Praise for Saving Teets

"Seldom do writings on cancer simultaneously twist our hearts in angst, joy, humor, tragedy, and wonderment—all by reading one page. In Saving Teets, *Carey Cornacchini's down-home writing has done just that, as she strips away the doom and gloom veneer of this insidious disease and offers a beacon of hope for anyone facing a life-altering crucible. Cornacchini is a modern-day superhero who has spilled her soul for all to see, and the world is a better place for her doing so.* Saving Teets *is a powerful lesson on how to remain courageous in the face of long odds, and is a book you must read, and will not soon forget."*

—**William Teets**, author of *Upside Down (One on the House)*, *Reverend Went Walking*, and *After the Fall.*

"In her poignant memoir, Saving Teets, *Carey Cornacchini artfully weaves together her experiences with thoughtfulness, humor, and profound perspective. With each turn of the page, readers are invited into her world, where resilience triumphs over adversity and laughter dances in the face of fear. Through her words, she offers solace, inspiration, and a reminder of the incredible power of the human spirit. This book is not just a memoir; it's a beacon of hope for anyone navigating their own journey through illness or hardship. Highly recommended for its authenticity, warmth, and unwavering spirit."*
—**Maureen Anderson**, MD.

"A truly intimate, inspiring and beautifully written story of how to use frightening health challenges to heal and transform ourselves, into greater states of wholeness."
—**Natalie Valentini**, L.M.S.W., A.A.C.S.W.

"This book was such a joy to read, I laughed, I cried, and I learned! Carey through her natural wit and wisdom gives us a glimpse inside her intimate journey conquering cancer, twice! Even more important, she shares her life philosophy that gave her the strength and courage to face the challenges head on."
—**Christina Cattell**

"Simply put, I loved this book. As an OB/GYN physician who has followed (too) many women through their cancer journeys, Carey's recounting of her own story will resonate with anyone touched by breast cancer. I found the book to be raw and real and funny and inspiring all at the same time. I laughed out loud at parts, then found myself teary at others. It was quite a ride. It was so engaging, I finished it almost in one sitting. By sharing her experience with such wit and wisdom, Carey will undoubtedly help countless others feel not so alone as they navigate through a breast cancer diagnosis."
—**Christine Matoian**

"I am an oncologist with over 30 years of caring for cancer patients like Carey. I can't recommend [Saving Teets] highly enough. She is a courageous woman who intimately shares her breast cancer journey. I laughed and I cried. And mostly I learned. Though I have journeyed with hundreds of patients over the years, her account reminds me how different and individual each journey is. Her book is a beacon of hope and understanding for patients, families and healthcare providers alike. Medical and nursing training spends a lot of time on disease and pharmacology, but relatively short on day-to-day patient experiences, the suffering and the joy, and how with a better understanding of these we can better serve our patients. I think I will get a couple dozen copies to share with our fellows in training and support staff. Families of newly diagnosed patients will find solace and guidance within its pages, through her raw honesty and unwavering strength, navigating the darkest moments with grace, leaving readers inspired and empowered. I was deeply moved, and I am sure most readers will be too."
—**Joe Anderson**, MD.

Saving Teets

A Comedic and Inspiring Story About Breast Cancer Survival

Carey Teets Cornacchini

GLOBAL WELLNESS MEDIA
STRATEGIC EDGE INNOVATIONS PUBLISHING
LOS ANGELES, TORONTO, MONTREAL

First Edition. Published by:
Global Wellness Media
Strategic Edge Innovations Publishing
440 N Barranca Ave #2027
Covina, California 91723
(866) 467-9090
StrategicEdgeInnovations.com

Editors: Waterford Writers Workshop
Illustrations: Red Emblem Design
Cover and Book design: Global Wellness Media

Saving Teets / Carey Cornacchini.—1st ed.
ISBN: 978-1-957343-27-3 (e-book)
ISBN: 978-1-957343-26-6 (Paperback)

Disclaimer

The information contained herein is not intended to be a substitute for professional evaluation and therapy with a health professional. If you are experiencing any health issues, you need to seek professional help.

This book is based on the author's personal experience and other real-life examples. To protect privacy, names have been changed in some cases.

Table of Contents

For Bob, for ALWAYS making me feel loved and cherished.

("I'm the winner!")

Acknowledgements

I'm immensely grateful for the following people who helped me on my journeys:

Every doctor, nurse, technician, and aide, who cared for me. You have shown me there are angels on earth.

Dr. Deborah Ruark, Dr. Yousef Hanna, Dr. Michael Walker, and Dr. Peter Chen for your expertise, dedication, and compassion.

Tina, my adopted sister, for visiting me one day, getting on my computer and saying—"Hey, let's set up a blog." Then keeping me on task to get my book published. I'd still be contemplating if you hadn't given me a gentle push.

My friends and family, who have supported me every step of the journey. Meals, cards, gifts, phone calls, visits—I **always** felt your love. One of the most precious gifts I've received from having cancer is the love and care from all of you.

My hairdresser and friend, Debbie, for giving me special moments to treasure in the darkest times.

My mom, Marilyn, thank you for your comic relief.

My father, Ritch, for showing me through his journey with the Big "C" that you must always find the humor. You are my idol.

To Cathy, Laurie and Toni, thank you for showing me that true friends are really life's treasures.

My siblings for their care. Ritchie, for his phone calls just to check in. My sister, Denise, for always being there for me. My sister-in-law, Renee, for helping me through chemo.

Auntie Dee and Uncle Jerry, thank you for your unwavering support, whether it be bringing meals, reading material, or just sitting with me during my tests and chemo treatments. We are blessed to have you in our lives.

To the Waterford Writers Workshop. Especially our leader, Bill Teets. (Can you believe I met someone with the same last name? What are the odds of that! And we're not related.) Thank you for your guidance, critiques and especially patience with this 'newbie.' My writing improved because of all of you.

To my fellow goddesses, Becky, Leslie, Heather, and Leslie. You ladies have given me unconditional love and support with no judgment. Navigating life with all of you has been a blessing.

To Natalie, where do I begin? You were my light in the storm. From the bottom of my heart, I sincerely thank you for guiding me through my journey of healing. Your unwavering belief in my abilities gave me the courage to face my fears and discover my inner strength and resilience. I am immensely grateful for having you in my life.

To my children, Nick (Molly), Anthony, and Riley. Thank you for being you. You gave me strength, love, hope, and comic relief. Through your words and actions, I always felt your love and support. I couldn't ask for better children (well, except for the phone calls that started with "Mom, here's the thing . . ." or "Is dad within listening distance?").

And finally, to wonderful Bob. You were my caregiver, chauffeur, confidant, protector, quite frankly you were my knight in shining armor. I'd love when we'd leave meetings with my doctors and you would say, "We can do this." I wasn't alone; we were in this together. My journey **was** easier because of you. You held me when I cried, laughed with me when we found the humor, let me rant when I was angry, and lovingly cared for me through every test, surgery, chemo, and radiation treatment. Thank you for being my partner, thank you for loving me, thank you for you. I love you!

Additional Materials & Resources

Access your Additional Materials & Resources
referenced throughout this book at
SavingTeets.com/bookbonus

Introduction

Wanting to remember my cancer journey, I began to journal during my first dance with the **Big "C"**. As a side note, you'll find most times I refer to cancer as the Big "C". My image is of a big *Cafone* (Italians will understand) a big, hairy, not very intelligent bully trying to throw his weight around. What a *buffoon.*

My first journey was a "drive by" version of cancer. Diagnosed on April 27, 2011, and I completed treatment by Jun 28, 2011. I "did" cancer in *60* days. Per my oncologist, I had a 97% cure rate. My cancer was a blip. I always felt embarrassed talking with other cancer patients about my journey because it wasn't difficult. What I experienced was *life-changing, not life-taking.* (One of many mantras you'll see throughout my book.)

In 2017, when diagnosed a second time, I knew this journey would be more intense. The Big "C" had decided one visit wasn't enough, *the bastard.* I would experience the full gamut this time: mastectomy, chemo, radiation, and all the side effects. The treatment would be more challenging (both physically and mentally).

My writing is more introspective. There are more dark days, fear crept in. Working daily at staying positive, being my own personal cheerleader; I gave myself pep talks. Most days I was able to find humor and gratitude.

I read something somewhere which sums up my second journey: *Cancer is not a death sentence, but rather it is a life sentence; it pushes one to live.* It's true. I am enjoying **living**.

Why a book? Though I love reading, I've never considered myself a writer. I started a blog (www.savingteets.com) on my second journey because I knew my cancer treatment would be more intensive. A blog would be an easy way to inform my family and friends about my progress. Talking about my cancer constantly was draining. But the main reason: writing helped me heal.

I would write when I felt sad, angry, overwhelmed, even on days when I laughed at it all. When I wrote, the worry, angst, sadness, and anger melted away. I could let it go. This book is just that—my blog of daily musings while on my journey. You'll read some redundancy in my writing, as I was constantly reminding myself to stay in the *now* and to find gratitude. *Daily affirmations.*

I received positive feedback from friends and family, who enjoyed my writing. While flattering, I often wondered if they were saying such niceties because they had to. After all, they *are* my friends and family.

But they began recommending my blog to people who were also on their own cancer journeys. I have talked to some of those women, and all said my blog made them laugh and find gratitude. When discussing gratitude with a woman one night, she texted me, thanking me for the conversation, she said, *"Tonight, my gratitude is you."* I broke down crying. Realizing my journey and writing helped someone, is a gift. Maybe the saying is true: *You were assigned this mountain to show others it can be moved.* —Mel Robbins.

I decided to publish my blog in hopes it will give someone a smile while they're on their own journey with the Big "C". Who knew I'd write a book that already had a sequel? Breast cancer, Take One and Take Two. Two for the price of one! I hope you enjoy reading about my story and all the gifts it gave me. May you smile and hopefully have a laugh or two while you're navigating your own journey.

P.S.: I'm in the process of researching breast reconstruction. Maybe I'll write a threequel (is that a word?) I can already see the title of my next book: "To Boob, or Not to Boob, that is the Question."

What's in a Name?

I think the title of my book needs some explanation. When trying to come up with a catchy title, I was stumped. Let's face it: When describing the breasts, the options are endless: tatas, the girls, bazoombas, headlights, etc. I found more than 138 slang words for breasts in an internet search, but nothing was grabbing at me. "Saving the Tatas," "Saving the girls," "Saving Second Base" had all been done. I wanted something original, something you wouldn't forget.

I really don't know why it took me so long to come up with the title *Saving Teets: One Woman's Journey with the Big 'C'*. My maiden name is Teets. Yes, you read it correctly—TEETS. I was destined to have a sense of humor. How can you not with a last name like that? If you don't have a sense of humor, you'll never survive. Try going to four different schools in four years with the last name of Teets (middle school till freshman year in high school—yep, those awkward teen years). To add to my teenage angst, my best friend's name growing up was Chris Szluk, so we were Szluk and Teets. Don't tell me God doesn't have a sense of humor.

Having that last name, you tend to be a target for quips. I do appreciate it when someone comes up with something original or better yet if I could come up with something witty to defuse the situation. I was working for Electronic Data Systems in the late '80s and it was my first phone call with a new customer. I knew I would need to supply my contact information. I still had a little bit of trepidation when giving out my name, always wondering what the reaction would be.

As the conversation ended, we began to exchange our contact information. I told my customer my last name, which was followed by silence, and then "Could you spell that, please?" I spelled it and heard him quietly say more to himself than me, "You did say that." I was holding back the laughter, and I could tell he was too. The poor man was trying to maintain some professional decorum.

I seized the opportunity and followed up with: "Yes, John, my last name is Teets. I work on Big Beaver Road and its off Exit 69." Decorum out the window, all I heard at that point was hysterical laughter. You can't make this stuff up. Real life is ironic. Why not just laugh along with it?

I wonder if having this last name somehow predestined me on this cancer journey. Who knows? I don't think anyone ever had the nerve to ask the origin of our name. Once my father wanted to see if we had a family crest. Can you imagine what that would have looked like? Truly, I have no idea where the name originated, but it has certainly made my life interesting. I even broached to my husband that maybe we should combine our names to Teetacchini or CornaTeets when we married. Honestly, the man really needs to get a sense of humor.

> *There are moments which mark your life;*
> *moments when you realize nothing will ever be*
> *the same and time is divided into two parts:*
> *Before this And After this.*
> —"Fallen"

BREAST CANCER
TAKE ONE
(2011-2017)

Diagnosis

And So, It Begins
April 16, 2011

It started with a routine mammogram. While on vacation in North Carolina, I got a call, my mammogram came back suspicious, and they want to take another look. Another look? What does that mean? This is a first for me since my tests have always been clear. I made an appointment for a follow-up mammogram and got off the phone. I'm in a daze, worst-case scenarios popping into my head, a black cloud is hovering over me. Now I'm anxious to get home.

It's early Saturday morning, as I'm driving to the Breast Cancer Center, I give myself a pep talk: *Keep calm and cool Carey.* After all, they only want to take a second look, right? A lot of women have to go back for second mammograms, and it turns out to be nothing.

When they call my name, I think *I've got this, I've been here before, I know where to go.* I not only go to the wrong side but walk right smack into the door. So much for coming across as calm and cool. If you're coming back for a second mammogram or have already had breast cancer, you go into a different waiting room.

Once I've changed into the requisite hospital gown, it's time for my mammogram. This time, they take X-rays in different poses than were taken last time. When done, I go to the waiting room, and sit in silence waiting to hear my future.

While waiting, one thing becomes crystal clear: Cancer doesn't discriminate. The diversity in the room astounds me. All shapes, sizes, ages, and ethnic origins are here. While very diverse from one another, we are all having a similar experience. We didn't "pass" the first go-round and are here for "another look." It's very quiet, no one is making conversation, all of us hoping for positive news. You can feel the tension. Even lost in my own thoughts, I feel a kinship with these women. They understand me and my reality. There is something powerful and comforting in that.

My wait is up. The pathologist wants to speak with me. *Great. This doesn't sound good.* I'm told there are calcification deposits in my left breast. He recommends a breast biopsy. Calcifications? Wait a minute, a breast biopsy? OK, I'll be honest—I didn't see that coming. I truly thought I was going to be told there was nothing.

The little black cloud hovering over me is starting to get larger. My anxiety level is off the charts. This is when, as I've termed it, the "*What If Syndrome*" tries to take over. I find myself going right to the scariest scenario. God forbid, I would have just said, "*Oh, they just want another look, it's nothing.*" Nope, I had to torture myself before I received any news. *What if* it's cancer? Which then led me to: *What if* it's a late stage? *What if* I need to have chemo? *What if* the cancer has gone somewhere else in my body? *What if...?* AHHH!!!

I have to force myself to stop my mind from running away from me. If I keep this up, I will have myself dead and buried. I was letting fear take over. When thinking about cancer, I never thought of the mental side of it. I'm struggling to get my mind under control. I mentally give myself a pep talk: "*Get it together, Carey, they just want another look. It's probably what he said it was—calcification.*"

Since this is Saturday, I will need to follow up with my internist on Monday for a breast specialist recommendation. Monday morning can't come soon enough!

> **I'm scared of the unknown future.**
> —Bethany Frankel

Anticipation
Sunday, April 17th

Days seem longer when you have a black cloud hovering over you. I spent the day trying not to think about my mammogram results yet failing miserably as I'm filled with nervous energy. I find myself counting the hours until I can call my internist. Come on Monday!

> *Being anxious is the worst feeling in the world.*
> —Enrique Englesias

All Set
Monday, April 18th

I have my phone in hand with the number pre-dialed, ready to push at 8:30 a.m. when my internist's office opens. I get through immediately and explain my results. They gave me two names of breast specialists. I choose Dr. Deborah Ruark, for her stellar reputation and because she's a woman. I wanted someone who could relate to me, someone who truly understood the female body.

I call her office as soon as I'm off the phone. My appointment is in two days, Wednesday, April 20th. I'm apprehensive but hopeful.

> *Trust yourself. You've survived a lot,*
> *and you'll survive whatever is coming.*
> —Robert Tew

Meeting with the Doctor
April 20th

I'm not nervous as I'm sure it's just calcification. My visit begins with an examination by Dr. Ruark. Little did I know it will be one of many examinations I will receive during my tangle with the Big "C".

She is kind, gentle, thorough, knowledgeable, and puts me at ease. She informs me there is an 80% chance what I have is calcification. *Eighty percent, those are great odds.* For the first time since this roller coaster started, I take a breath. The black cloud is getting smaller. Now

I just have to get through the biopsy. One more step and I'm finished. *Woo-hoo!*

> **Don't count your chickens before they hatch.**
> —Thomas Howell

The Big Breast Oil Change
April 20th

It's the day of the biopsy; my appointment is for 8:00 a.m. I have a sleepless night, looking at the clock every hour and wake up tired. Okay, I'll admit it, I'm scared. I don't have a phobia about needles, but there was something about the combination of breasts and needles that leaves me terrified. The unknown has my stomach in knots.

The clinical description of the biopsy:

*For a Core Needle Biopsy, the doctor uses a hollow needle to take out pieces of breast tissue from a suspicious area the doctor has felt on exam or has seen on an imaging test. The needle may be attached to a spring-loaded tool that moves the needle in and out of the tissue quickly, or it may be attached to a suction device that helps pull breast tissue into the needle (known as a **vacuum-assisted core biopsy**).*

My description of the biopsy:

My breast was getting an oil change!

Once at the hospital and the preliminaries were completed, I'm brought into a room with a large rectangular table. I have a **huge** confession to make here: I didn't read the information given to me about the procedure. I know shame on me. Let's just say there was some denial going on. I just didn't want to deal with it.

As I'm taking deep breaths, the procedure is explained to me. I'm to disrobe (just the top), climb onto the table, lay face down, then place my breast into a hole that's in the middle of the table. Once in place, the table will be raised, the doctor will sit underneath me and perform the biopsy. I was partially listening, as I was busy worrying about the dreaded shot. Did I just hear her correctly? I said, "Excuse me, but did you just say I was to put my breast through a hole on that table?" She explains the procedure again. She did say that. Say what?

Several things pop into my head: First: Will the hole be large enough to accommodate my huge breast? Second: Just how high will this table go? But the predominant thought and image I can't get out of my mind: *OMG—my breast is having an oil change!*

All types of images flash through my mind. Is the doctor going to motion me onto the table like the attendant does at the oil change shop, using hand motions to get me into the right spot? "No, Carey, move a little to the left, now come forward, slower, slower . . . that's it. Stop." I picture myself lying prone on the table, with my breast hanging down through a hole, the doctor in blue overalls with a dipstick in his hand. Could this get any worse?

AND about that time, it does. In walks the doctor and, just my luck, he's young and gorgeous. Think McDreamy—get the picture? I turn to the nurse and say, "You've got to be kidding me!" She laughs, pats my hand, and says, "I know dear, I know." I guess it somewhat helps she understands my pain.

At this point, fear and trepidation left my mind and were replaced with one thought and one thought only: "Why in the hell didn't I lose those 50 pounds I've been meaning to lose?" Yep, the day is heading downhill fast. Do the irony gods have to rain on me today? I mean really, not only am I exposing myself to a room full of strangers, laying prone on a table with one breast through a hole—I get to have Dr. McDreamy do the procedure.

Once my shock has slightly worn off, I see McDreamy looks quite young. Great, Doogie Howser is going to perform my biopsy. I ask the doctor his age and he replied, "I'm in my 40s." I look at him again (you know the look you give your children when you know they're lying) and he says, "OK, just 40, but I did a fellowship at Harvard." At least Doogie Howser is well trained, so I feel more at ease.

As I'm climbing on the table (a dignity stealing torture device), I wonder if the hole will be large enough. I get up as gracefully as I can (I'm sure that was a sight) and place my breast through the hole. Lucky me! The person who developed this device makes sure it's adjustable and my breast fits just fine.

Face down on the table, my breast down through a hole, my head to the side, holding the nurse's hand I can't help but think not only am I worried I might have cancer, but I also must go through **this** procedure to find out. The word dignity doesn't seem to fit here.

The table is raised. They adjust my breast and put it into a vice-like grip—think of getting a mammogram lying down. When I'm all set, the doctor rolls under me in his chair—OMG—I'm mortified.

The part I've been dreading happens. My breast is numbed. I felt a tiny prick followed by a stinging sensation which lasts about five seconds. Whew! Dreaded part over and not too terrible.

"Doogie McDreamy" explains every part of the procedure. He tells me there will be one point in the procedure where I will hear a popping sound. He will warn me ahead of time, not because of any pain I will feel, but so I won't jump at the sound. This is when he places the tube into my breast to begin pulling out the samples.

Once completely numbed, he forewarns me. I lay perfectly still. Pop! I felt tugging while he was pulling out the samples, but there was no pain. Several clips are put into the area for future identification should the biopsy come back as cancer.

The procedure itself doesn't last long. Band-Aid on, I'm ready to go home. I ice my breast for the rest of the day—no worse for wear. I learned some important lessons today: (1) read the information given about procedures (2) apprehension is sometimes worse than reality and (3) I need to stay in the present moment and stop letting my mind wander. Little did I know this is something I will need to embrace in the future.

> *Beware of apprehension, for it kills hope, weakens*
> *actions, and brings about worry.*
> —Iman Ali

The Wait
April 27th

Biopsy complete—now the '**wait**' begins. I hate the wait. It's adding insult to injury. Waiting for the phone call which could change my life. The statement "Life can change on a dime" resonates with me. I want it to ring, and I don't want it to ring. If it doesn't ring, I can ignore it for a little bit longer, but at the same time, I want to know. This is so difficult.

> *Patience is not the ability to wait but the ability to*
> *keep a good attitude while waiting.*
> —Joyce Meyer

Results—AKA Life Just Turned on a Dime
April 28th

It's two days after the biopsy, I was in the middle of making dinner when I get the call. Amazing how I'll always remember exactly where I was when I get the news.

When we first met, my doctor explained 80% of calcification is not cancer. It seems I was the 20%. My diagnosis: ductal carcinoma in situ—basically, cancer was in my ductal glands. An appointment is set for tomorrow to discuss options.

Hearing the word "cancer" turns my world on its axis. It's Thursday, April 28, 2011, and **I HAVE BREAST CANCER**. My worst fear has just been realized and I'm numb. I can feel that black cloud consuming me, and my world seems a little less bright. *There is cancer inside my body. This is really happening.* I knew deep in my gut this was a life-changing moment for me. Life from here on out would be different. Where will this journey lead me?

I don't have time to deal with my news. I'm a mom, and Anthony and Riley are home. I have to leave within the hour to drive Riley to dance practice. But first, I need to tell my husband. What to do? As I didn't want either of my kids to overhear my conversation, I walk outside to call Bob with the news. I'm surprised how calm I am when I do this. I don't cry but am sad.

He listens intently, asking questions I can't answer and then making sure I was alright before we got off the phone. In all the years he was traveling for work, it would be the first time he didn't come home on a Thursday night. He would be home tomorrow in time to see Dr. Ruark. Husband told; I need to focus on my daughter. We have to leave soon. I can't react to my news. Once I understand my diagnosis, treatment options, and prognosis I will tell my children.

We arrive at the high school for her dress rehearsal. I'm feeling out of sorts but still no tears. Well, the gods decided they would help me out on that front. While walking out of the high school, I trip, get airborne and fall onto the pavement in front of several students. I fall hard—shoes come off, purse flying, jeans ripped, elbow scraped—I'm sure it was a sight to see. An epic face-plant.

I need help to sit up and it takes a few minutes to get my bearings. I'm literally seeing stars. Someone has told my daughter, and she comes running out in a panic to see what happened. Great, just what I need! I keep a stiff upper lip while limping to my car and tell her I'm fine. *Come on, really? I just get a cancer diagnosis and now this?*

Once in my car, I call my husband. He answers and the dam breaks. I'm hysterical and sobbing. In addition to the embarrassment of swan diving in front of the entire dance group, I've skinned my knee, and my arm is throbbing. Poor Bob, he can't understand what I'm saying and since it was just a few hours after the cancer call, he thinks I've gotten more news on my diagnosis. He obviously knows I'm hysterical and says, "What? There's more cancer?" I sob out: "Nooooo! I fell and skinned my knee and it's bleeding." There was a long silence then: "You're crying about that and not the cancer?"

Looking back, it was a release of tension and to be honest, even though I'm battered and bruised, it was good to cry. It helps me immensely. Another lesson learned: *You don't always have to be brave. A good cry helps every now and again.*

I phone my sister to tell her my news. She wants to come over and talk. I want to be alone. I **need** to be alone. There is no "right way" to handle having cancer, each person handles it differently. For me, I had to regroup and process this information by myself. I didn't want to offend anyone, but I need this solitary time. This was the first step of caring for me, something I haven't done in a very long time.

Sitting in my rocking chair with my every present dog, Winston, on my lap, I feel powerless. I *don't* want to have cancer. I *didn't* choose this. *God, I'm so scared.* The longer I sit, the more frustrated I feel. I have no control over what is happening to me, and I desperately want control. After a long time in the silence, I realize I need to challenge myself with what I can control, *my attitude*. Once my mind went to that place, calm began setting in. I was beginning to feel some of my power coming back.

My attitude will decide what kind of journey I will have. No matter what the outcome of this wild ride, hysteria isn't welcome. Serenity and optimism are my new mindset. I *will* have a peaceful journey.

> *Peace—it does not mean to be in a place where there is no noise, trouble or hard work. It means to be in the midst of those things and still be calm in your heart.*
> —Unknown

The Plan
April 29th

My appointment with the breast surgeon is at 1:00 today. I spend the morning watching the royal wedding of Prince William and Kate Middleton while waiting for Bob to come home. (Come on, who doesn't love a royal wedding?) Mindless diversion.

Once he arrives, it's just the two of us as the kids are at school. Sharing alone time together is what we need. We talk, cry, hold each other and gather our strength to start this journey.

Armed with my planner to take notes, we head to my appointment. I'm feeling low when we arrive. While in the waiting room, we see a family who has just found out their loved one has advanced stage breast cancer. Seeing their fear and pain, I say to Bob we have nothing to complain about. We are blessed. I'm reminded there are so many other people who are having a much harder journey than I am.

The first thing Dr. Ruark said to us, "I have the best possible news to give you today." What a wonderful gift. Her words washed calm over me. The black cloud is disappearing.

I have ductal carcinoma in situ (DCIS), cancer of the ducts, non-invasive, low grade, slow growing with a 1% chance of spreading. *Wowee! Wow! Wow!* I'm at Stage 0! I didn't even know there was such a thing. Treatment options were a lumpectomy followed by radiation or a mastectomy. During the lumpectomy, Dr. Ruark will remove 5 cm from my breast (*trust me, it won't make a dent*).

At Stage 0, a mastectomy didn't seem like an option I wanted to take. Though to be honest, removing these gargantuan breasts and starting over did pass through my mind. Think: I could see my feet, no worries about them smothering me while I slept, clothes would fit nicer. Decision made; I opt for a lumpectomy followed by 6 weeks of radiation. We leave feeling somewhat relieved and ready to tackle the next step.

Even though I'm Stage 0, my mind still goes into overdrive. I wonder what caused my cancer. Is it possible it's somewhere else?

Would she be able to get it all? Will surgery hurt? Radiation? AHHH! My mind was reeling. Once again, I had caved into the fear of the unknown. Will I ever learn?

> *Don't let fear win.*
> —Unknown

Getting the Tools
April 30th

Physically, I feel fine. Mentally, not so much. Unglued would describe my mental state. I know I need tools to help me navigate this; it's too overwhelming. I'm not the only one going through this cancer journey. How can I help my family deal with this when I feel so lost?

I've been taking a development class every other Wednesday for 10 years plus with the magical Natalie. Together with four other amazing women (Becky, Leslie, Heather & Leslie), we navigate life together. Nothing's off the table for discussion. We talk, laugh (a lot), meditate, and grow together. It's a safe and supportive environment where we can share without judgment. Natalie has led us on this journey of growth, and I can't thank her enough.

I turned to her for help. The first thing she says to me: "Stay in the present moment. Stay in the now." Letting my mind wander to the "What Ifs" won't serve me. *I certainly, was learning that one the hard way.* This is one of the most important lessons the Big "C" is teaching me. It ties in with *Enjoy Your Nows.* I need to flow and just be in the present moment.

Natalie also reminds me to remember to **Breathe**. Yes, I know you are all saying, "Duh?" We all breathe but the majority of the time it's shallow breath. She reminds me a deep cleansing breath will help calm and center me. Breathe in *Gratitude* for the past, hold *Grace* for the present and release while *Grounding* for my future. When I start to panic, stop and take three deep cleansing breaths applying that mantra.

17

And finally, she reminds me to find the gratitude in what this journey will give me.

Stay present, remember to breathe, and find gratitude. Three important components to my healing journey. Thank you, Natalie.

> *One day at a time. Head up, take a deep breath. Stay strong.*
> —Surf Girl

And One More Component—Humor
April 30th

In addition to staying present, breathing and gratitude, I've decided I *need* to find humor in my journey with the Big "C".

I was lucky enough to have an amazing father. My dad had several serious medical issues in his life and through all of them maintained a fantastic sense of humor. He survived all the odds given to him so when he was diagnosed with melanoma, we thought it was just another bump in his life path. He was invincible in our eyes. Unfortunately, he was already in Stage 4 when diagnosed. He opted to not have any treatment, wanting to enjoy what time he had left.

He was diagnosed in April, and we would lose him in September. For six months, I witnessed my father live his life in joy. We have a large extended family and every night they would converge at the house, gather around the dining room table, and reminisce. Dad would sit in his lazy boy chair and laugh with all of us. At one point, I said to him, "Dad it's like you're attending your own wake." He laughed and said, "I know; how lucky am I?"

One day, Bob and I were with him, and he began discussing his funeral. "No box wine at my wake, get the good stuff," he said. He told us he was going to be cremated. Then said, "When your mother dies, my ashes are going to be put in her casket, so what I want you to do is make sure my ashes are on top." I asked why, he started laughing and said, "So I'm in control for the rest of eternity." I was still reeling from that tidbit when he got serious and said to me, "Carey, even during this, you have to maintain your sense of humor. Humor is what gets you through."

It was the last lesson my father would give me and now that I'm on my journey with the Big "C", I realize it's the most precious lesson I could have ever received. Thank you, Dad, for showing me how to live my life with humor.

> *I never would have made it if I could not have laughed. It lifted me momentarily out of this horrible situation, just enough to make it livable.*
> —Victor Frankl

Telling My Children
May 1st

I've met with my surgeon and had a "tune up" with Natalie to help me process my diagnosis. I want to be mentally prepared when speaking with my children. Even though I'm still coping with my news, I have to figure out how to help them navigate this. I was the one with cancer, but as a parent it can't be just about me.

I'm in the early stages with a great success rate. They need to understand things are going to happen in life which are out of your control; it's how you handle it that matters. Attitude and gratitude are everything. *God, I am dreading this.*

I've given a lot of thought to my approach. The goal is to make sure they aren't scared and understand this isn't a death sentence, but a bump in the road. I tell you; my speech was Oscar worthy.

We plan to tell them on Sunday night after Riley's dance competition. Our oldest, Nick, was home from college but had to head back on Saturday so we told him then. Nick never gets flustered. Calm, cool and collected, that's him (a future pilot skill in the making). He handles it with the usual aplomb. He understands the prognosis and seems alright. I'll still worry about him, it's a lot to take in.

On Sunday night, home from the dance competition, we asked Riley and Anthony to sit with us. I'm really worried about them, both extremely sensitive souls. As we sit down, I begin my 'epic' speech. I immediately choke up. Looking at their faces, I can't get the words out. I turn to my husband with pleading eyes, hoping for his help. This turns out to be a *really* bad idea. He looks at me with panic in his eyes, turns to the kids and blurts out, "Your mom has cancer!" *OMG, are you kidding me?*

Suffice it to say, that snaps me out of my crying. Not quite the delivery I was aiming for, but it nonetheless got their attention. (*Another lesson learned: Let your husband know your practiced speech beforehand in case he has to pinch-hit for you.*) My melancholy gone and knowing if I let him speak anymore, my kids would be more than scared, I began talking to my children.

With the two of them listening, I explain how I'm extremely lucky the cancer was contained and caught in very early stages. My daughter immediately asks: *"Am I going to get it?"* My response is "No." She then asks: *"You mean like the breast cancer Mimi had last year?"*

If anyone has teenage sons, you will understand what I'm about to tell you. Anthony, who has been listening intently but has not said a thing yet, pipes up and says: *"Mimi had breast cancer last year?"* OMG, he seriously asked this? No reaction to my news, but he looks incredulous his grandmother had breast cancer the year prior. I couldn't help it, I burst out laughing. Thanks for the comic relief, Anthony, and once again proof that teenage boys do live in their own world. Don't you just love him? Kids informed of my diagnosis—Check. Now on to informing my mother.

Everybody needs someone to make them laugh when they think they're never going to smile again.
—Unknown

Telling My Mother—or the World
May 3rd

I've told my siblings about my diagnosis but hesitated to tell my mother. She was having minor surgery and was apprehensive. Right before her scheduled surgery, she had been ill on vacation and went to a clinic. She was told by a quack doctor she had cancer. She flew home immediately and saw her own doctor. He reassured her she was fine, but this minor surgery was making her very nervous. I plan to tell her after her surgery.

That was *one* reason I didn't tell her, but the real reason was I knew it would be shared with the world once she found out. Telegraph, telephone, tell Marilyn—LOL. I love my mother, but she can burn up those phone lines. Whenever she goes on a trip, the first thing she packs is her phone book. Get the picture?

I decided when I was diagnosed this would be my journey to handle my way. I truly didn't want a cast of thousands involved for several reasons—the main one being it takes a lot of energy to have cancer, let alone having to discuss it with everyone.

Every time I told someone, I had to relive the trauma of it and let cancer suck a little more energy from me. I wanted to focus my energy on myself and my immediate family. In some ways, it was the first time I had really made it all about me. Another big lesson learned from having the Big C: *Take time for you, take care of you, love you.*

She came through the surgery with flying colors, and everything turned out fine. My sister and I brought her home, and I figured after her nap and a nice dinner; I'd tell her. We just came in the door and my sister looks at me and mouths "TELL HER" I start laughing and my mother wants to know what's so funny. I tell her my diagnosis, what I have done thus far, dates of my surgery, etc. Her first response: *"Oh my God, and you hosted Easter dinner knowing this!"* (With her upcoming surgery, I ended up hosting Easter for 30 people). She was more shocked about that than my cancer diagnosis. Thanks for the comic relief, Mom. Once I finished, I follow with *"Let's not make a big deal about this. I'd like to handle this quietly."* I leave and laughingly tell my sister to keep a lid on her.

At home a few hours later, I call my sister, chuckle, and say, *"Please tell me she's behaving." "Too late,"* my sister laughs. *"The phone book was out before you left the driveway—she's gone from A to Z. The phone lines have been burning."* LOL, yep, so much for keeping my diagnosis quiet.

> ***Telegraph, telephone, tell Marilyn.***
> —Carey

Surgery

Time for Surgery—Take One
May 14th

I received a phone call from the hospital letting me know my surgery time, what preparations I need to do and requesting additional information. Why is the additional information always my weight? Really? Must I tell every stranger what I weigh? *Honestly!* I'm told to wear something easy to get into, like a jogging suit. A jogging suit? Do I even have one of those? Now I'm worried about what I'm supposed to wear. Maybe that's OK because I'm focused on looking good when I arrive at the hospital.

I only want my husband and sister with me; too many people would have been stressful. I opt for the same attitude I had with my labor and deliveries. My mantra: suck it up princess, this time tomorrow it will all be over.

My nerves are frayed from the anticipation. I didn't get much sleep last night. I meditated and prayed in those dark hours, thought too much, forgetting at times to stay in the now, wondering what the next day would bring. My mind on overload.

I put on something similar to a jogging suit that I found in the back of my closet along with my new underwire bra (more about the bra later) and head to the hospital. The drive to the hospital is quiet. I'm holding on by a thread, afraid if I talk, I'll cry. Working hard to stay in the moment.

Arriving at the hospital, the first thing they have me do is step on scale! Really? In addition to being scared, I have to get weighed? (*Life is not fair people.*) I'm taken to a private room and the wait begins. *Breathe, Carey.* Reading my new Kindle while waiting calms me.

While being prepped I'm told I will be taken to the mammogram area where a wire will be inserted into my breast. This will help the surgeon locate the cancerous area. I'll be numbed for the procedure but fully awake. *Oh yay! More needles!* (Keep Breathing Carey.)

A kind volunteer takes me up to the waiting room. While I sit in a wheelchair with a blanket around my shoulders, I feel so lost. No one could do this for me. I'm the one who has to go through treatment and recovery. This is the lowest point in my journey so far. Fear, anticipation and the reality of what is about to happen are hitting me.

There may have been other women in the room. I don't remember. The television was on, but I couldn't tell you what was playing. All I feel in this moment is gut-wrenching fear and sadness. Tears are welling up in my eyes and I'm trying so hard not to cry. I've been brave for everyone, but I'm not feeling very brave right now. *God, I'm so scared.* I close my eyes and breathe. I take deep-from-the-toes breaths and begin to feel calm setting in.

I'm wheeled into a room which has a mini mammogram machine. Normally, patients stand during the procedure, but once again my giant tatas come into play. The tech decides to have me sit because my breasts will fit into the machine better. *Yay!* Finally, a benefit for the large tatas. Still nervous and filled with anticipation but joking with the tech about the tatas and asking about her has eased my fear a little bit. This is something I tend to do with medical personnel. I want to know who is working on me. Knowing something personal about them makes it less clinical. Joking with them makes it bearable. I find the more I can laugh at everything the better I feel. *"Laughter is an instant vacation."*— Milton Berle.

The door opens and who should appear? Doogie McDreamy. Really? Will I ever get a break? I chuckle and say: "You again? You're a nice guy, but I was hoping to never see you again." That gets a laugh. Tension gone. He begins the procedure. My breast is put into the machine and once again numbed. The apprehension is less with the needle this time as I knew what to expect. He begins. I can feel the wire going in, but there isn't any pain. The procedure takes no time at all. Wire in place, I'm taken down to wait for surgery with my family.

It's time for the surgery. I'm given twilight sleep—3—2—1—OUT. The procedure lasts 45 minutes. A 2½-inch-size lump is removed along with six margins. (I'm sad to say taking out that amount still doesn't shrink the tata.) I wake up in recovery crying. I think it's a release it's over. Dr. Ruark says everything went well, and she will call me within the week with the results. They released me to go home with a prescription for Vicodin to help with pain.

On to the bra story: Just a word to the wise when selecting a bra to wear to surgery; don't pick the cutesy underwire bra. Choose a bra that closes in the front. While Bob got the car, Denise was helping me maneuver the tatas into the bra. It wasn't pretty. I'm sure my sister had never seen anything like that before. I think she's scarred.

One thing I realize, check your dignity at the door. You will be exposing yourself to countless strangers. Having a sense of humor will get you through it. *Trust me*. I did it, I survived the surgery; now the wait begins.

> *A well-balanced sense of humor is the poll that adds balance as you walk the tightrope of life.*
> —William Arthur Ward

The Decimation
May 18th

The first few days home from surgery, I find my favorite friends are frozen peas and Vicodin. The peas are used for the incision area and the Vicodin is for any pain. I don't feel bad, but I take the Vicodin to stave off any future discomfort. I'm not a huge pill popper. I rarely take an aspirin and was petrified of Vicodin. I'm such a wimp, I think I'll become addicted. I will admit, though, they work.

My doctor has suggested taking a stool softener with the Vicodin. I've never had any trouble in that area, but being the rule follower that I am, I send my husband out to get some.

Now here's something very important to remember: When sending one's husband out to get a stool softener, make sure he reads the label. The boxes for both laxative and stool softeners are green. You see where I'm going with this right?

I'm in my faithful rocking chair and even though I haven't experienced any side effects from the Vicodin, good little soldier that I am, I decide I'd better take the stool softener. My husband, the ever-present caretaker, gives me the pill.

About a half an hour later, I think I'm giving birth in the bathroom. I yell to my husband there's something wrong, my daughter can hear me in pain and wants to know if everything's alright. *I think I'm dying.* An hour later, cleared out, cold sweat gone, my coloring coming back, I go to the linen closet and look at the box. **Laxative**. I have no words. I've just been decimated by my well-meaning husband. Of course, he has me swear not to tell anyone about his blunder—yeah, right!

> *God Bless him, he tried.*
> —Carey

Thoughts While Waiting
May 19th

What I find hardest throughout this journey is the WAITING. You have the tests, surgeries, and procedures and then you have the dreaded wait for your results. The results which will tell you what path you're going to take. Your life is in the balance.

While waiting to hear if the margins are clear, if I let it, my mind can take me places I don't need to go. I'm trying to follow Natalie's advice to stay in the moment. Thinking ahead and worrying about the different scenarios won't help. Logically, I know this, but fear is trying to work its way in. I have to work very hard at staying focused and positive, and I find when I do, I'm much calmer.

The diagnosis of cancer leads you on a soul-searching journey. It is a life changer. What I used to think was important no longer is, anger at small things is a waste of energy. I'm learning to find gratitude daily. I read this somewhere and it became my reality:

> *When you intentionally divert your attention to gratitude and appreciation, you're not only feeling better, you're literally changing the content of your thoughts, and, in so doing, you create the opportunity to change your reality.*

I am determined to find gratitude in my journey with the Big "C" no matter what results I receive.

> **Gratitude is a powerful catalyst for happiness.**
> —Amy Collette

Life Just Turned on a Dime, Again
May 20th

Dr. Ruark calls, it's not quite the news I want. Five of the six margins are clear, but one margin came back with a different kind of cancer— Invasive Lobular Carcinoma. When I hear the word invasive my stomach drops. Up to this point, I've been told it's contained.

I've got two types of cancer in the same area. I have more cancer. Seriously? Not the call I was expecting. *Breathe, Carey.*

She goes on to explain treatment: Another lumpectomy with removal of lymph nodes. The good news: the lobular carcinoma is 1.1 milliliters. Miniscule. I'm lucky—a great pathologist caught it. I'm not happy to have another lumpectomy, but I quickly check myself and think about the woman I saw that day in Dr. Ruark's office who was at Stage 4. This is just another bump in the road on my cancer journey.

> **The bump in the road is just an opportunity to overcome challenge.**
> —Unknown

Breast MRI—Taking a Closer Look
May 25th

Dr. Ruark has scheduled me for a breast MRI. This procedure will show if there is any additional cancer in my breast. Even though I'm worried; I'm having no apprehension about the procedure. My thoughts: No problem, I'll lay back and sleep in a tube. I've got this.

Wrong! I've concluded there is something with breast cancer and machines with holes in them. Being totally prepared to lay on my back, to my surprise I'm told I must lay on my stomach with, you guessed it, my breasts through a hole. Patty (who has two boys and a girl, in case you were wondering) gives me an IV and I proceed to lay face down. Once again, I'm worrying whether the gazoombas are too large for the holes. Thank God they fit.

She hands me ear plugs, tells me the procedure will take 25 minutes, and suggests I close my eyes and make up to-do lists in my head. I try to do that but eventually go with the old standby, saying Our Fathers and Hail Mary's. What can I say? I'm Catholic. It's amazing how one's faith pops up in the unforeseen moments.

I eventually start praying to the loud beat of the machine. Kind of a rap version of the Our Father and the Hail Mary. *Whatever works.* MRI completed; I'm told I'll get the results later today. Once again, I'm astounded how quickly this is moving. True to form, Dr. Ruark calls. The news tips in my favor for once. No other cancer—*Whoop! Whoop!* I finally feel like I can take a deep breath.

> ***All in all, good news and a good day.***
> —Michael Morales

Well, I Thought I Was Calm
May 27th

My surgeon wants to meet with me to discuss my upcoming lumpectomy. While waiting for my doctor, her physician's assistant

(PA), comes in to explain the procedure. Radioactive dye will be injected into my breast before surgery so the hot spots will reveal which lymph nodes need to be biopsied. Oh yay, more needles in my breast. Can't wait—not.

That was enough information for me, but she continues and says she's had patients say this was extremely painful. TMI, Theresa. I'd rather been surprised. There was no worry for this surgery since I'd already been through it. So much for that! Fear and anxiety are now occupying my mind. Focus Carey, stay in the NOW. Breathe.

> *Realize that the present moment is all you have.*
> —Ekhart Tolle

Breast Lumpectomy—Take Two
May 30th

I'm semi-calm for today's surgery. Calm, because I know the logistics of the surgery, nervous for the dreaded injection. In my gown, my IV inserted (ouch), I wait for the radioactive dye injection. (*Taking deep breaths here.*) The doctor comes in carrying a little black box with a lock. Looking at the box, it sinks in, he's going to inject radioactive dye in my body. *Why does treating cancer have to be so toxic?*

Needing to feel calm, I immediately start grilling my visitor. Where was he from? Where did he get his degree? The usual fifth degree questions. He's a nice Slavic man who immigrated in the '80s. The dreaded injection doesn't hurt, all I feel is the prick of the needle. I think my prayers to my deceased father asking him to help me with the pain worked. *Thanks, Dad.*

As the doctor leaves, he tells me to jiggle my breast to help spread the dye around. Does he really know what he's asking? With this gargantuan breast if I do that, it may never stop. Sitting and 'jiggling' my breast waiting for surgery, I think about all the wasted energy on worrying. When will I ever learn?

I'm wheeled into surgery and the next thing I know I'm in recovery with Denise telling me excitedly my lymph nodes were clear. *Double Whoop! Whoop!*

I wake up to a burning sensation. The doctor explains to me she had to go through the original incision hence the burning. In addition, there is a new incision under my arm where the lymph nodes were taken. This surgery is more painful than the last but still bearable. I'm sent home with instructions of ice and Vicodin.

I learned another lesson today: When driving someone home from breast surgery, bringing the family Jeep is not a great idea. You feel every bump on the road. Put it this way: Riding home groggy from surgery, holding my breast with two hands (yes, it takes two to hold that puppy up) was not my idea of a joyride.

It *is* fantastic news about the lymph nodes, but I still must wait to hear the results on the margins that were tested. The wait begins, *again!*

> *Worry is a waste of time. Good and bad things will happen in life. You just have to keep living, and not stress over what you can't control.*
> —Not Salmon

It's Good News!
June 3rd

Thank goodness the wait isn't long, and the news is great—*no more cancer.* All margins are clear. I'm doing a happy dance. *Whoop! Whoop!* Now on to treatment.

> *Today it hit me—Today is a good day!*
> —Unknown

Radiation—AKA Zap Time

On to Radiation Treatment
June 9th

The additional treatment for my breast cancer will be radiation. After researching, I opt to have Dr. Chen for my radiation oncologist. He has a stellar reputation. Unfortunately, he is the choice of many and is booked out. By not being able to see him, the timing of the radiation would mean I would have to miss my daughter's national dance competition. I don't want to miss it.

Praying again to my deceased dad to help me. (His track record has been pretty good during this journey.) I call the office to see if they can squeeze me in. When they ask Dr. Chen, he looks at my address and notices I live four doors down from his parents' old home. He agrees to see me tomorrow. *(Thanks, Dad.)* I'm filled with gratitude.

> *Express gratitude for the greatness of small things.*
> —Richie Norton

The Decision
June 10th

After hearing from everyone that radiation is a breeze, my nerves are fine as we drive to the hospital. Once we arrive at the cancer center, I'm taken right back. First thing they have me do… step on a scale. Really? A scale at the front desk? Who does that? Not only am I going to have to strip and show my tatas, but I also have to weigh myself at the front desk? *Oh happy days.*

Weight taken, put in a room, it's time to do the 'usual,' which, for a breast cancer patient, strip from the waist up and put on a hospital gown with the open part in the front. Dr. Chen's internist enters and begins to explain about a new clinical trial, *Contura Brachytherapy.* There are certain criteria which must be met to qualify for the trial. You have a diagnosis of Ductal carcinoma in situ (DCIS) and your surgery has to be within a certain timeframe. I meet the qualifications. The Contura device looks like a balloon with four prongs. The balloon is placed inside your chest, where the cancer was, with the four prongs outside your body. During treatment the prongs are hooked up to a machine which administers the radiation seeds to the affected area. The seeds are swished around and brought out. The procedure is done twice a day for two days, then treatment is complete.

My initial reaction is NO. The thought of my breast being butchered again sends me into a tailspin. *No, no and no!* He leaves and Dr. Chen enters. We discuss the neighborhood for a few minutes and then he talks about the clinical trial.

My husband pipes up: *"Sure, we'll do it."* My response: *"Just a minute, Baba Louie, last time I looked it was my breast he was talking about and there is no 'we' in surgery."*

Knowing my husband, his logic was 2 days vs. 6 weeks that much quicker to put this all behind us. I ask more questions and get more comfortable with the procedure. Dr. Chen gives us time to ourselves. I think about the pros and cons—pros win out (2 days and helping with a clinical trial), I agree to the procedure.

> *Plan your execution—Execute your plan.*
> —Unknown

And Yet Another Surgery
June 14th

The Contura device will be implanted into my breast today. Waiting in my prep room, *surprise,* in walks the same nurse from my previous surgery. Seeing her feels like home. Then I think; have I been here so much I'm getting to know the staff? *Yikes.*

There are no nerves today, having just had surgery I know the drill. Twilight sleep given, up an hour later, Contura in place; I'm ready to go home. Instructions: keep my bra on and no showering.

While getting ready to go home, my nurse says, "You are so lucky you had the device surgically implanted. My friend had hers put in in her doctor's office and it was unbearable." Once again, I'm reminded how lucky I am to have such a compassionate doctor.

Before I leave, they set an appointment for a CT scan tomorrow. The scan will show if the device is in correctly. One more hurdle completed—closer to the finish line. *Whoop! Whoop!*

> *Life may put a hurdle in your way, but life also gave you legs to jump over it.*
> —Jesse Byer

Just an Everyday CT Scan—or so I Thought
June 15th

Today will be one more hurdle closer to the finish line and I can't wait to get it done. There is no pain with the Contura, though my body knows it's there. The quicker I get to treatment, the quicker I can get this out.

Going through so many tests and procedures, I've realized something. During these visits I dissociate from myself, like I'm floating above my body watching. I find I must detach to not feel embarrassed when having to strip and go topless. It was difficult doing this when I had a younger body. Now? *Mortified.*

The other thing I do, when undressing, I always, **always**, fold my bra and underwear and place them underneath my clothes. They are going to look at my most private parts, but God forbid they see my bra and underwear.

Gown on and sitting on the table when the technician approaches, I go into 'detach' mode and open my gown. I sense something is off when he averts his eyes. He says, *"Ah, we can cover you up for this procedure.*" OMG, I've just flashed the guy. Could it get any worse? I soon find out; it is going to get worse.

While on the table, he's in another room running the CT scan. I hear him say, *"Hmmm. Let's take another look at this. Let me call someone."*

"What?" I ask, *"That doesn't sound good. What does that mean?"*

After a few people are called in to look at my scan, the head of the radiation department comes to me (*it must not be good if they've called in the big guns*). He tells me the Contura is leaking fluid. It seems I have the one, in the thousands of devices, which is faulty. It's the first time in the history of the company this has happened. *Are you kidding me?*

My oncology radiologist, Dr. Chen, is on vacation. The doctor asks me if I want to remove it, quit the clinical trial, and do the standard radiation protocol. My answer is no, but if I'm honest here, it was partly because I don't want to have the device removed by strangers. Someone else touching my breast threw me into a panic. *I know, suddenly, I've become territorial?* It sounds crazy, but my breast (and me) had had enough abuse. Quite frankly, I certainly wasn't thinking rationally because it eventually it had to come out. I just knew in that moment I didn't want it removed. They release me to go home, and I'm told I'll hear from my breast surgeon later.

When Dr. Ruark calls, I find out my luck gets even better, all representatives are in Las Vegas for a convention, and I won't be able to get a new Contura until next week. Yep, one week living with the faulty device in my body. *Lucky me.* I must continue to wear my bra 24/7 with no showering. Ever take a bath with a bra on? *Fun times.*

This time when I receive the new unit, the procedure will be done in Dr. Ruark's office not under twilight sleep with surgery. Thinking about what the nurse told me about her friend's experience, has me scared. *Breathe, Carey.*

> ### You can't avoid mistakes and bad luck.
> —Mikhail Tal

Next Steps
June 16th

Dr. Ruark wants to check on me and discuss next steps. At my appointment, I express my concern about having the procedure done in her office. I tell her what the nurse told me about her friend's experience. She senses my apprehension and instructs me to take two Vicodin an hour before I go to her office. We leave with an appointment set for June 22nd. *Keep breathing Carey.*

> **The chaos doesn't end, you kinda just become the calm.**
> —Nikki Rowe

Out With Old, In With the New
June 22nd

Today's the day of the procedure and fear is taking over. I take the Vicodin, hoping it helps my stress level. Arriving at the office, the company's representative greets me and says he's going to observe. Really? Isn't it bad enough I have to have this procedure? Now he's in there with me? *Breathe and Detach Carey. Breathe and detach.*

After letting him know that I was not happy to meet him, he says, "Hey, there's good news. We're not charging you for the faulty device." *You're kidding me, right?*

My doctor knows my apprehension about the injection into my breast. She uses a very small needle, and I don't feel a thing. Everything numbed, there was no pain only pressure when she is replacing it. *(I really have a great doctor.)*

Once again, the anticipation was much worse than the procedure, though having the rep there wasn't ideal. Faulty Contura out and new one in. Jumped another hurdle. *Whoop! Whoop!* On to the CT scan tomorrow, fingers crossed hoping it's good news.

> *All of us have bad luck and good luck. The man who persists through the bad luck—who keeps right on going—is the man who is there when the good luck comes—and is ready to receive it.*
> —Robert Collier

CT Scan—Take Two
June 23rd

I'm back in the hospital for another scan, hoping this Contura is not faulty. The room is filled with people. Seriously, that many people are needed to see if the device is working correctly? Geez, why didn't they just sell tickets? Couldn't the tech just give them the news? I feel like a specimen. Breathe and pray Carey. Nothing a good Our Father and Hail Mary can't help.

The scan is complete, *finally* good news. This Contura doesn't leak. I'm cleared to start treatment and will be done three days before I leave for my daughter's dance nationals. *Whoop! Whoop!*

The Club

When I walk into the waiting room after the scan is done, the intern working with Dr. Chen is waiting to hear my news (obviously, she didn't get the memo about attending with the cast of thousands). I give her a thumbs-up and, she starts clapping quietly.

That was nice, but what is amazing were all the ladies sitting there in their different stages of cancer, who started clapping for me and telling me congratulations. They don't know me or even what my good news is but want to let me know they are happy for me. Getting good news, any good news, is a miracle in itself.

When you go through this, you see all types of people who are on their own private journey, but all share one common bond—**hope**. *Hope* the outcome will be positive. *Hope* if it isn't, you will have a peaceful journey. *Hope* the journey, whatever it is, will be one filled with abundant love. I am now a part of the Big "C" club, and the club was letting this member know they were behind me. I am humbled.

> *Once you choose hope, anything is possible.*
> —Christopher Reeve

Treatment, Finally!
June 27th

My first treatment is at 9:00 a.m.; with my second treatment at 3:00 p.m. I will be doing this for the next two days. I'm apprehensive but am told there is no pain. Hooking me up by my prongs to a machine? I'm just unsure how this is going to work.

I arrive and change into the uniform (hospital gown). I'm brought into a room with a large cone-like machine. While I hop on the table, Tang introduces himself. He's responsible for positioning the machine which will be administering the radiation.

It must be precise, and Tang takes his job *very* seriously. He is moving the machine millimeters at a time to get it in the right spot. Though I'm a little frustrated he's taking so long, I'm grateful he is so methodical. After all, he's dealing with radiation and, more importantly, me.

Once in place, my four prongs, which were hanging out of my breast, are hooked up. And it begins, I feel a pulsing but that's it. For a half an hour pellets of radiation are pumped in through the balloon, basically swished around the area where the cancer was, and taken out again. It was painless.

I'm back at 3:00 to spend some more time with Tang, who's definitely not a talker. Two treatments down, two to go.

> *I may not be to the finish line yet, but I'm on my way.*
> —Anonymous

Finished
June 28th

It's my 25th wedding anniversary. When I married 25 years ago, I imagined my anniversary would be spent on a beach drinking a pina colada, not hooked up to a machine treating breast cancer. My children are with me for this momentous occasion. Bob is out of town for work.

We're in the waiting room when Dr. Chen comes in and engages with my kids. He is so kind to my children. He even remembers my oldest is training to be a pilot and discusses it with him.

The nurse arrives, it's time. One last treatment, and I'm done with this journey. As I head off, my parting word is 'Behave.' They are 22, 19 and 16 but old habits are hard to break. In the room, Tang, again, takes his time lining me up exactly right and the process begins.

As I lay for the procedure and feel a light pulsing through the tubes into my breast, I'm at peace. I reminisce about my journey. I think about my husband and kids and how this has impacted our lives. This has given us a new appreciation of life, for each other. "*I love you*" is said more often and meant when it is said. There is happiness in little things. We have come out of this a stronger and more loving family.

I never had anger or asked, "why me?" *Why not me?* I'm just one of millions to experience this. (1 in 8 will have breast cancer). With my diagnosis, I have it easy in the grand scheme of things. I am Stage 0/1a and qualified for a clinical trial. I've been given a 97% cure rate. I got to meet some incredible people during this journey who have touched my soul. I've grown and learned more about myself than any other experience in my life. Why not look at this in gratitude? Life is too short for anger.

I'm done! I leave the treatment room and hold my kids. Having them there meant everything to me. Those hugs are the sweetest of my life. I am filled with love. The nurses come out to clap and present me with a gift. Treatment is complete. *Whoop! Whoop!*

We decide to go to dinner to celebrate. (*Any excuse to get out of cooking*) Sitting at the restaurant, I call my husband, and for the first time in a long time I can take a deep breath. While we eat, we talk about our journey with the Big "C"—well Riley and I talk; the boys per usual give me one-word answers. I think they grasp it. I get my confirmation when we're home, and I look at Facebook. Anthony posted this: *"With the right attitude you can get through anything."* He understood; they all understood. Life happens and what you do, when it does, makes all the difference.

> *Gratitude and attitude are not challenges; they are choices.*
> —Robert Braathe

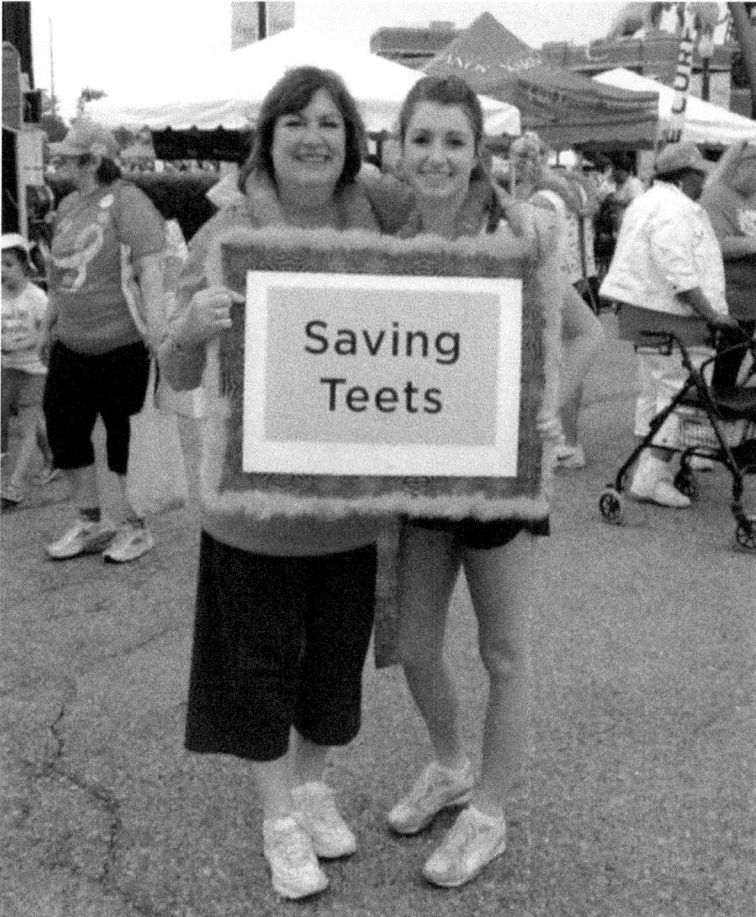

Five-Year Anniversary

The Shadow
March 12, 2016

I was ecstatic to have my five-year anniversary. I received my mammogram results, filled with joy, I was compelled to write.

Me and my shadow . . . I've had a shadow with me the past 5 years. A shadow I notice not all the time, but I know it's always there—hovering around me not quite ready to let go. Though I didn't want it, this shadow has taught me many things over the past 5 years: how life can change in an instant; that you may not be able to control something, but you can control your reaction to it; that fear tries to be your best friend when life is uncertain and doesn't want to let you go; how finding faith, hope and a sense of humor gets you through. It showed me the precious gift I have with my family and friends. It helped me see I no longer have time for toxicity in my life and to embrace the positive. It led me to Reiki and the gift of administering to cancer patients. I learned I can be tested and look back on that test with gratitude. Gratitude for the growth and abundant love it gave me.

I received the test results from my 5-year mammogram yesterday. So, to cancer who has hovered in the shadows the last 5 years, there in the back of my mind, every time I went to a doctor appointment, had a mammogram, took a pill, felt a twinge of pain, or when fear invaded my head—I'M DONE WITH YOU! Five years clear. I value the lessons I've learned and the growth I've received, but now it's time to start life fresh without the shadow. Life has just gotten brighter.

Little did I know that the shadow had never left me but remained to take me on another journey.

BREAST CANCER TAKE TWO (2017–2018)

Because having it once wasn't enough!

Second Diagnosis

Here We Go Again
March 24, 2017

Every January I know it's time to schedule my annual mammogram. I passed the five-year mark and am heading into six years clear so there are no worries for the test. My doctor has ordered a 3D mammogram. Since it's 3D and because of circumstances in my life, I'm unable to get an appointment until the end of March.

While getting ready this morning, I noticed Riley is nervous about my test. To ease her worries, I asked if she wanted to come with me. She does. I'm fine with this as she needs to understand there is nothing to fear. I'm excited to have the 3D mammogram as I think it means my breasts wouldn't be pressed in the machine's vise-like grip.

So much for wishful thinking. My breasts are once again subjected to the squishing process. The only difference is the tech takes more pictures. I guess they thought during the last set of images, since I didn't have to hold my breath, they were giving me a bonus.

Afterward, the technician brings Riley in the room to see the machine and my breast images. While showing her the images—she asks the technician, "My mom's okay, right?" The tech says, "Yes, everything looks fine." (*Appeasing my daughter, I'm sure.*)

As we're leaving, Riley asks me what happens next.

"If everything is fine, I get a letter confirming it's normal. If not, I get a phone call asking me to come in for a second look."

"What if you get a phone call?"

My response, "I'll get another one and handle it."

On to shopping and lunch, a perfect way to end a mammogram day.

> *Today is the first day of a brand-new journey.*
> —Unknown

Another Look
March 28th

The one sentence no cancer survivor wants to hear is, *"We need you to come in for another look."* It's been six years since I had breast cancer and I've diligently gone to all my mammograms. Being on a clinical trial, I went every four months for a few years, followed by every six months and then once a year. They've all come back clear.

I'm in my car in the parking lot at Kroger when I get the call. *They've seen something and I need another mammogram.* I'll be honest, it's not what I expected. You see, I think I'm done with cancer. I had my dance and I've learned and grown from it. I really don't want another journey.

When the person who called me started to go through what I needed to do for the second mammogram, I stopped her and said, "This isn't my first rodeo, I know the drill, I've had breast cancer before." Her response: "I'm so sorry." She doesn't need to feel sorry for me. This is just my story. It's my path, and it will lead me where I need to go.

Ending the phone call, I put my head down on the steering wheel and deep sadness overcomes me. My poor breast. I stop. This isn't honoring me. Panic isn't welcome. I immediately ground myself and get centered. My first thought was to go home and lick my wounds, but cooler heads prevail, and I do my grocery shopping. Getting food and eating sounds like a good idea—*OMG, I think I'm a stress eater.*

When you have survived cancer, it's still there in the back of your mind. Every twinge, every pain, every time you go for a mammogram, you wonder: Is it back? I passed the five-year mark. I thought I was home free. Deep down, I know in my gut I will have a second dance.

But for now, while waiting to have my second mammogram, I will try not to worry and work at staying present. *And* I'll probably eat.

> *Worry is like a rocking chair: it gives you something to do but never gets you anywhere.*
> —Erma Bombeck

Let's Try This Again
March 30th

At the Cancer Center to have my second mammogram, I think about how confident and at ease I was just a few weeks ago after my previous one. Now they want another look. I'm trying to be upbeat, but my track record with follow-up mammograms isn't that great. Nerves are taking over. *Breathe, Carey.*

I do the drill and put on the body flattering gown (not) and walk into the waiting room. As last time, I'm astounded at the diversity in the room. Reminding me again how cancer doesn't discriminate. Everyone is like me, waiting to have another look. Some of us have already had the dance, others waiting to hear if they will be on their first Big "C" journey. Everyone sits in silence; all lost in thought.

While getting my mammogram, I make small talk with the technician. As she's placing my breast in the machine, or 'vise' as I like to refer to it, I mention I've already had cancer in this breast. She says: "Aren't you sorry you didn't have it removed?" *Really, lady?* I'm here to get a second look and am obviously on edge because I've been down this road before, and you say that to me? I swear some people don't think before they speak. My response to her: "I never look back."

Mammogram complete followed by the call. They have found calcification, and I will need to have a biopsy. The journey has begun again. *Keep Breathing, Carey.*

> *Nothing in all the world is more dangerous than*
> *sincere ignorance and conscientious stupidity.*
> —Martin Luther King, Jr.

Big Breast Oil Change—Take Two
May 9th

There's no need to read the instructions to know what the biopsy entailed. I've already had an "oil change." I opt to have it done at the

Royal Oak campus since the last time I was at the Troy campus. Maybe a change of scenery would give me better luck.

My nerves are fine, I just want the numbing injection over with. My doctor is lovely, she's energetic and kind. The nurse working with her is Russian and one tough cookie. She is forcibly clear with her instructions; they sounded more like orders. The room setup is different at this hospital. Their table doesn't lift, it's already at the correct height. (I feel a little less like I'm having an oil change.) I have to climb up a small ladder to get on the table. *Oh yay, they're making me work for it.*

I begin climbing, being careful not to trip while trying to hold the gown in place. God forbid they would see my tatas. I have no idea where that thought came from, they were working on my breast so why I was trying to hide them is beyond me. *Why does every test involving breast cancer make me lose my dignity?*

Once in place, the doctor begins. Numbing done. *Whew!* We talk during the procedure. We're discussing all types of things. Everything but cancer. The conversation keeps my mind off what is happening.

It's time for the pop. When the doctor inserts the tube to extract the calcium deposits; I'm to lie very still. My nurse has decided to help me out in that department. She lays her body on top of my back to ensure I don't move. Didn't see that *coming*. Popping sound happens and I feel a tugging. Breast oil change complete—now the **wait**. *Breathe, Carey.*

> *On particularly rough days when I'm sure I can't possibly endure, I remind myself that my track record or getting through bad days so far is 100%.*
> —Anonymous

The Big Easy
May 12th–15th

We're going to New Orleans to celebrate our friend Ken's 60th birthday. It's going to be a huge celebration. I'm hoping to enjoy the weekend and not focus on the results.

Our son Nick says, *"Hey, I don't have to work, and I can deadhead on the same flights as you. I think I'll join you."* (Deadhead—free flights for pilots)

My response: *"I don't remember inviting you."*

He responds with—*"Uncle Ken's kids asked me."*

I contacted the hotel and change the reservation to two queen beds since Nick will be joining us. Being a poor struggling pilot, I can guess who will be paying. We're fine with it. He's sacrificed a lot for his career. We're happy to bring him with us.

We have a great time in the Big Easy. Exploring, dancing, eating, and imbibing. Just what we needed. While we're walking through the French Quarter, we arrive at the St. Louis Cathedral. I *need* to go in. After lighting a candle and kneeling to pray, my emotions get the best of me, and I cry quietly. I cry for what's to come. Praying for wisdom, strength, and humor.

Lost in my thoughts, I forget my friend Meg is kneeling next to me. She asks me what's wrong. I'm hesitant to tell her as Bob is the only one who knows. I trust her. She is kind, caring and gives me comfort. Just what was needed at that moment. I leave the church feeling at peace. I've turned it over to God. What will be will be. I have a feeling I'm in for another grand adventure.

> *Inner peace begins the moment you choose not to allow another person or event to control your emotions.*
> —Pema Chodron

The Call
May 19th

Friday, May 19, 2017, and I have cancer **again**! Dr. Ruark calls to tell me. My first response: "OK, let's talk next steps." Not OMG, its cancer, or immediate crying. No. I knew I had it so let's get on with it. We talk a little bit. I'm not sure what we said. She makes an appointment with me for Monday. I tell her to have a great weekend, but I'll be honest, I don't remember what time my appointment is because all I hear is cancer—**AGAIN**.

Bob comes in and I break down sobbing. A tiny part of me was hoping I was wrong. I **really** don't want to do this again. The timing sucks. There is never a good time for cancer, but Nick and Molly are getting married in August. Riley is scheduled to study abroad in Barcelona. Anthony is finally in his dream job. We're all happy. F**K! Yes, I said F**K! It's the only word that fit the moment.

I apologize to Bob saying I'm so sorry to put him through this again. His response? "We fought it together before, we'll fight it again." He has an appointment and doesn't want to leave. "I'll be just fine," I tell him. I *want* to be by myself to process the news. I know, like I did last time, I need to be alone.

After he leaves, sitting by myself, holding Winston, I'm lost in thought. Having him on my lap gives me a sense of calm and I desperately need calm. I don't think this is going to be as short a journey like the last time. My gut is telling me I'm in for a wild ride; that I will be challenged physically and mentally like never before. Can I stay in gratitude? Will I be able to find the humor? Will my body be up for the treatments? *God, what am I in for?*

As I learned before, it doesn't serve me to ask questions which have no answers. *Fear is not wanted, stay in the now, Carey.* I need to change my attitude. There's a choice to make; have a pity party for myself or suck it up princess and deal with it.

I decide to suck it up and *dance*. I go to the kitchen and turn on the tunes and dance my heart out. Earth Wind & Fire's 'September' is put on repeat several times. I find myself smiling and feeling a little free. Bob calls me at one point. I see his number and I hold the phone to the music. "Don't Worry Be Happy" is playing. Yes, we need to not let worry or fear take over. We need to be grateful and happy just where we are.

I had met with Dr. Ruark before the biopsy, and we've discussed next steps if it is cancer. I want both breasts removed. I'm done with this set. Bob's response? "I've always been a leg and ass man myself." *God, I love this man!* We make the decision as we did last time to hold off on telling our children until we have a plan in place. Meanwhile, I'll keep dancing.

> ***Sometimes music is the only thing that takes your mind off everything else.***
> —Tiny Buddha

The Plan—Take Two
May 22nd

Since all I heard was 'cancer' when Dr. Ruark called to give me the news, I have to call her office this morning to confirm my appointment. Bob will be in Dallas for the week and can't accompany me to my 12:45 time. I'm fine by myself, but my doctor has requested someone come with me for an *extra set of ears*. Denise joins me. We agree she will take notes.

Entering the room, the nurse asks if I want Denise to be in the room for my examination. *Uh, no.* We're close but not that close. I receive exams from Theresa, the nurse practitioner (NP), followed by Dr. Ruark. One of many I'll have on this journey.

With examinations done, we move on to the game plan. I'll be honest, I naively think I will have a double mastectomy with no chemo or radiation. Just cut out the cancer was my mindset and have reconstruction. I'll be the old lady with perky breasts. *There is a positive here—LOL.*

The biopsy showed invasive lobular cancer cells. Dr. Ruark thinks its Stage 2 but will not know until she operates. The cancer is in two different areas and is slow growing. She recommends a mastectomy of the left breast, followed by chemo and radiation. Lymph nodes will be tested to see if my cancer has spread. *Damn, I'm in for a battle.*

I want a *double* mastectomy, but Dr. Ruark doesn't want to remove both; she wants me to begin treatment as soon as possible. Having both breasts removed increases the odds of infection or complications which could prevent me from receiving treatment. She explains the sooner a patient receives chemo and radiation, the greater the odds of survival. I'm not happy, but I understand. Out of everything she has said, what devastates me most is having chemo. My son is getting married in August. I want to have hair for the wedding. *Double damn!*

While I diligently take notes and ask questions, my doctor stops and says, *"Are you alright?"* I'm confused until I look over and see my sister crying. Denise blurts out, *"Do you want me to take notes?"* OMG—LOL! *"Nope, don't worry, I've got this."* I love my sister and I found it hilarious. The comic relief was welcome, but also another reminder cancer doesn't just affect me. It touches those around me.

As I'm leaving, my doctor says she loves my attitude and energy and wishes she could give it to other patients. Here's the rub: I have no control of this, **none** whatsoever. The only control I have is my reaction. I've done cancer before; I get how it tries to grab you and fill you with fear, but if I'm going through this again, it's not going to own me. There *must be* gratitude and humor.

The office schedules a PET and bone scan for the following Thursday. Once again, I'm hit with how fast everything is moving. As we head to the elevators, I choke up and say to my sister, "I really want to have hair for Nick's wedding." I want to enjoy every aspect of his wedding, not deal with this, dammit!

Before I leave, I have to get some blood work done along with a chest X-ray. *Shit just got real; this is **really** happening.* As we're heading home after, the hospital calls. They didn't take enough blood. I have to come back. *Great.* This is not starting out well.

After more blood is drawn, we decide to go dinner. *Can you say stress eating?* While figuring out where to eat, Nick calls on his way home from the airport. He's a pilot with a crazy schedule, so I have to grab him when I can. I ask him to come to the house to talk.

Life has just turned on a dime once more. I have to tell my children I have cancer. Something I never thought I would ever have to do again.

> *You may not control all the events that happen to us, but you can decide not to be reduced by them.*
> —Maya Angelou

Telling My Children—Take Two
May 22nd

Learning from my last dance with the Big "C", I waited to share my diagnosis. By giving myself time to digest the information and allowing the grief, it enabled me to feel centered and ready to tackle my next journey. When telling my children, I wanted to be empowered, not lost.

My first thought when receiving the diagnosis: *"I have cancer again!"* which was quickly followed with*"OMG, I have to tell my children I have cancer again."* As a parent, this is one of my worst nightmares. I'm devastated.

Since Bob is in Dallas this week, I will tell them by myself. This is fine with me since the last time he pinched hit for me it was a disaster. (LOL) When I arrive home, Nick and Riley are waiting for me. Anthony is at work until 9. I want to tell them together, but with Nick's schedule, I have to do it now. (*God, I really don't want to do this again.*)

Tearfully I explain my diagnosis. When going through the tentative plan, Riley cries silently and Nick becomes stoic. I apologize to Nick saying I'm sorry to have this now when it's supposed to be one of the most joyous times in his life. He looks at me and says, *"What are you sorry for? Don't say that."* I tell him, *"I won't have hair for your wedding."* His response: *"Who cares? You'll have two more weddings."* My daughter stays quiet. I let them know we're just facing another bump in the road; we'll navigate through it together. Nick

53

leaves and I receive a text from him: *I love you and we'll get through this mom.*

Riley and I plan a mindless evening. She convinces me to watch the "Bachelor," only after I convince her to watch "Dancing with the Stars." Mindless diversions are needed right now.

Nick texts again and invites us over to Molly's for dinner. We decide to go, we'll watch our mindless shows when we get home. On the way, Riley has a huge meltdown and cries, *"This is not fair. You've already had cancer."* I remind her how life isn't fair; that everyone has something. We'll all learn and grow from this and like last time it will give us many gifts. We just have to look for the silver linings. We enjoy our meal and forget about life for a while. Just what we needed.

Anthony comes home, and I go into his room to speak with him. I don't find it any easier getting the words out. His initial response: *"Well, that sucks!"* Anthony asks me why I didn't remove my breast the last time. With the stage I was in and the cure rate I was given, it didn't seem necessary. I can't look back. I can only move forward. Children told, now on to tell the world.

> *It is bad news, but we just have to get on and deal with it.*
> —Alan Phillips

Telling My Mother—Take Two
May 22nd

There is humor in having cancer. Grab it when you get it, folks. It helps ground you and brings you back when *fear* wants to take hold. My mother *always* helps me find the humor.

While I was telling my children, my sister went to tell my mother. The last time I had cancer, and she was told, her response was priceless. This time her response was no different.

When Denise told mom, she blurted: *"Why couldn't it be you?"* (*Say what, Mom!?*) She did follow it with, *"Why couldn't it be me?"* Then asked why it wasn't happening to my other sister this time. I guess she's an equal opportunity sacrificer. (Is that a word?)

Her response was truly about her angst of my having cancer again. She just said the first thing that popped into her mind out of her love and frustration. Thanks for always making me laugh, Mom.

> *Every time you find humor in a difficult situation you win.*
> —Avinash Wandre

The Healing
May 24th

Every Wednesday, there is a healing service at the St. Bonaventure Chapel at the Fr. Solanus Casey Center. Over the years I have prayed over his casket. I've even chaired several fundraising events for the center. You're surrounded by peace when you're there; it's a place of miracles. Today, I decided to attend with Riley.

I'm a lapsed Catholic—okay, I'm a Creaster (Christmas and Easter)—but I've never lost my faith or spirituality. I pray more now than when I was a 'regular.' I believe in the miracle of prayer and the healing it provides. My last experience with the Big "C" taught me faith isn't just a word but a true part of my life.

The church is filled to capacity. Everyone hoping for a miracle. It's a very moving service, the brothers pass along a microphone and allow people to verbalize their petitions. Their stories show me mine is just one of many, and there is so much to be grateful for. The service ends and people line up for a healing.

While Riley and I wait our turn, I notice the brother doesn't ask any questions but instinctively knows what blessing to give everyone. What we are witnessing is profound.

When it's my turn, the brother holds my hand. I hold Riley's; other people placing their hands on me. He places the relic on my forehead and tells me to feel the healing light going through me. My body feels heat. I have never felt a more powerful presence of spirit.

Riley steps up to receive her healing. I have my hands on her, as do several people around us. The brother's healing and message: calm her mind, let go and feel peace. The ceremony is overwhelming for her, and she is crying. I'm sad, but at the same time happy to share this with her, and grateful to witness her experience faith in action. A memory I will hold forever. *Cancer* gave that to me. I leave empowered with the holy spirit in me. My journey is one of peace and acceptance.

> **Faith, it doesn't make things easy, it makes them possible.**
> Luke 1:37

More Tests (Oh Yay)
May 25th

I'm at the hospital to have a PET and bone scan. Riley is with me; she *wants* to be here. Auntie Dee and Uncle Jerry join us. I'm glad they are here to sit with her as I have no idea how long the tests will take and don't want her to be alone.

The first test is a PET scan. I have an hour to drink FDG (Fluorodeoxyglucose), the most administered radiopharmaceutical in PET scans. The taste is godawful and knowing there's a timeframe puts pressure on me. They give me a sucker to help offset the unpleasantness. I start a rhythm: take a drink, suck on the sucker, take a drink, suck on the sucker. *Thank God for the sucker.* I finish on time and am back in the waiting room to wait an hour while the radioactive compound distributes throughout my body. *Oh yay, more chemicals.*

While waiting, Uncle Jerry explains what will happen during my tests, as he has had the procedures before. During the PET scan, I will be in an MRI-type machine lying completely still. He said at one point, I will feel heat from my groin to my throat. *(Heat from where to where?)*

My mind immediately goes into overdrive. *How hot? How long will it last? Bring it back, Carey. Stay present. Breathe.*

The hour is up and I'm off. I put on a gown (seems to be a prerequisite for every test) lay down on the table and am moved into a tube. The test begins. While lying there, I go to my fallback and begin to recite the Our Father and Hail Mary. The prayers bring me calm. The technician speaks to me periodically and warns me of the heat to come. And it does. Zing! Streaks of hotness from my groin to my throat just like Uncle Jerry said. Thankfully, it lasts less than 10 seconds. Test done. One down, one to go. On to the bone scan.

Since mine is the last test of the day, and the office is empty, the technician lets my family in the treatment room with me. Uncle Jerry opts out. I don't blame him; he's already been through these tests.

The technician explains that during the test, I will lie on a table and the machine will move over me. It will be just inches over my body. *Okay, then, can you say claustrophobic?* This is the last test, but it may prove more taxing.

Auntie Dee stays near the door, Riley stands where I can see her. The test begins, and the machine starts over my lower body working its way up. I close my eyes and breathe. *And* the prayers begin. One hour later, I'm done.

These tests are important. They will show if there are cancer cells anywhere else in my body and help determine my plan of action. I've finally wrapped my head around having breast cancer again, will I be able to handle it if it's elsewhere? It's Thursday night, right before Memorial Day weekend. I won't get the results until Monday or Tuesday. Will I be able to stay present while waiting? Damn it's going to be a **long** weekend.

After eating dinner with Auntie Dee and Uncle Jerry, Riley and I head home. On the way, I ask her about the test she watched. She tells me she stood close so she could surround me in the white light of protection. I've always told my children I surround them in the white light of Christ, and now my sweet, giving daughter is doing that for me.

Yes, what I'm going through is horrendous, but look at the gifts it's giving me.

> **Gratitude is a memory of the heart.**
> —Jean-Baptiste Massieu

And Yet Another Wait
May 27th

I'm in the valley today and feel out of control. Waiting for my test results, my mind is not staying present. Friends and family know about the tests, and even though they mean well, I get constant text messages and phone calls asking me if I've received any news. Lesson learned: Don't tell people about the tests until **after** they're done.

Overwhelmed, I call Natalie and she helps me get out of my head. It's odd to say, but I can handle having breast cancer again. Having it somewhere else in my body, that's another story.

Unsettled my entire body is being examined, I start focusing on every pain and ache. Could it be cancer? Between the texts, phone calls, and my wandering mind, I find myself in the middle of the "What If" syndrome. Will I ever learn?

Natalie reminds me about the results: "I don't know." That's all. *I just don't know*. Leave it at that. Conjuring up scenarios doesn't serve me. Stay in the **now**.

I give myself a pep talk. (*Suck it up, princess; get on with life and stop wallowing*). I decided to keep busy; exercising, cooking, and shopping (who doesn't like a little retail therapy?)

While desperately trying to stay in the now, I do the unthinkable for me, I weed my garden. Me, the woman who kills every plant within a 10-mile radius, weeding. *Talk about desperate.*

I'm knee-deep in the garden, Bob and Riley are watching me. Their looks go from amazement to hilarity. It's the first time they have seen me weeding. Yes, I said the first time. I don't garden—**ever**. I look at the weeds as cancer trying to infect my flowers. Well, to hell with that! I become a madwoman, grabbing the offensive cancer weeds tugging with all my might. *Take that, you little bastard!*

I become obsessed with making sure every single weed is gone from the garden. Bob keeps trying to get me to stop, saying he will get it later. That's not happening on my watch. I continue to weed with a vengeance. I do wish I had listened though when he told me to put on long pants because my legs are covered with mosquito bites when I'm finished. Nevertheless, I prevail. Every single weed is eradicated from the garden. I felt like a superhero for saving my plants from the 'cancer.' I have a sense of peace when done.

I make a list of what I need to prepare before surgery.

1. Purchase a La-Z-Boy chair to sit in during recovery.
2. Go to a breast cancer specialty store and get supplies to help with my healing.
3. Make meals to put in the freezer.
4. Get a massage.
5. Get a manicure.
6. Get my hair cut and colored.
7. Load up my Kindle with books to read.

Hyper-focused, my plan of attack is comforting to me, and gives me back some of my lost control. I was taking my fear and **F**ocusing my **E**nergy to **A**lter the **R**esult. Cancer is a mind game, and today I am winning. Out of the valley.

> *Always remember your focus determines your reality.*
> —George Lucas

Still Waiting!
May 30th

I've planned a busy day. My goal is to keep myself occupied so I don't focus on my test results. I begin by going to a breast cancer store. I need to order shirts with pouches for the drains to wear after my mastectomy. I ask a lot of questions, wanting to know what will happen to me, what to expect. (*Here I go again with that control thing.*) Each person tells me what I already know but don't want to hear: There is no *'set'* way. Everybody's recovery time is different. I could have the tubes draining anywhere from three days to three weeks. *Lovely!*

I ask about the steps after the surgery and am told I will have to wait four to five weeks to get fitted for a prosthesis. If I begin chemo in August, it's suggested I buy my wig in early July. (I wonder what I would look like as a blonde?) Plans made to help me navigate my new normal, I move on with the rest of my day.

After lunch, I still haven't received my results. I had the tests on Thursday—it's now Tuesday—the longer the wait, the more my nerves take over. I've kept myself occupied all weekend, kept up my mantra about the results, "*I just don't know,*" but by today, my mind is having difficulty focusing.

I registered with Beaumont My Chart, so I would get immediate notification of my test results. I'd like to think I'm somewhat brave, but when I saw my results were online, I couldn't bring myself to look. What I desperately waited for all weekend, now petrified me. I sat staring at the screen.

Bob came in, and I finally have the courage to log on. We sit together, but I can't click on Test Results. I break down and say, "*I'm a coward, I'm afraid.*" He holds me saying nothing, just giving me his loving energy. More centered, I look at the bone scan results. A little arthritis, but all is clear. I breathe a little better but can't bring myself to look at the body scan. *I just can't do it.* Bob sees I'm at the breaking point, so he doesn't press me.

I leave to get my haircut and massage. My rationale is if it is bad news, I want a few more hours of peace. I know I have cancer, but in this moment, it was only in my breast.

I enjoy getting "puffed and fluffed," committing to memory the sensations. I ask my hairdresser, Debbie, "How many clients have you had who get their hair cut and colored for a mastectomy?" We laugh. Laughing felt good. At least my hair will look great for the surgery. Hair done, on to my massage.

Dr. Ruark's office calls as I'm driving. Her assistant says she wants to see me tomorrow at 10:30 to discuss my surgery. I ask if she has my test results. She responds, "They're on top of your chart right here, the doctor will discuss them with you tomorrow." That doesn't sound good. *(She wants to discuss it with me? What does that mean?)* I realize then I can't wait until tomorrow. I need to look at the results when I get home. *Damn it.*

I'm at a stop sign concentrating on my breath, deep breath in, deep breath out, calming myself, when the office calls again. *What now?*

The assistant says, "I realize when I got off the phone with you that I may have misled you about your test results. I spoke with Dr. Ruark, and she told me to call you to let you know your test results are clear; she will only be discussing your surgery with you tomorrow."

What a gift she just gave me. I knew from the last time I had cancer, when you receive good news, it is truly a gift. I am filled with gratitude. I tell her she has made my day. I immediately call Bob and sob when I tell him the great news. We're both laugh and cry at the same time. *I'm so blessed!*

When I got home after my massage, Bob was in the driveway. I jumped out of my car, we hugged, laughed, and cried some more. We stop hugging and do a happy dance on the driveway, waving and swinging our arms like little kids. *Pure bliss.* We text our children to let them know the happy news. *Relief.*

Riley soon comes home, and I greet her with a hug. She sobs in my arms. *(She gets it.)* She knows how precious this information is. I get a text from Nick, who tells me he loves me and is happy about the results. Anthony hugs me when he gets home from work, and says, *"Finally, good news."*

As difficult as this is for all of us to deal with, it also brings us closer. A switch has been turned on; we *get* what's important; *Love.* Pure and simple LOVE. I'm surrounded by it and am grateful.

> ***When we focus on our gratitude, the tide of disappointment goes out, and the tide of love rushes in.***
> —Kirstin Armstrong

Moving On
May 31st

At my appointment, Dr. Ruark explains the surgery will take at least two hours. She will remove my breast and do the pathology while I'm on the table. I will be staying overnight and go home the following day. It doesn't seem like a long hospital stay, but insurance companies believe the stay is long enough. *I wonder how many of those who have set the timeline have had a mastectomy.* Armed with the information I need; Bob goes to get the car.

Since I'm in the hospital where I volunteer, I want to say goodbye to the people I have worked with over the past three years. I visit the integrative medicine department and receive hugs, words of encouragement and support.

Next stop the infusion center, where I have administered Reiki, to say goodbye to the nurses. I tell them about my cancer and find myself choking up when I tell them I'm to have chemo. The warm caring smile I receive from one of them touches my heart. They say very lovingly they'd love to take care of me.

How surreal is this? The place where I have given Reiki to so many to ease their burden of chemo is where I will be in the next few months. Will I be able to handle this as gracefully as others have? I want to have my chemo here so I can feel at home. This place has been my piece of heaven for three years. It has allowed me to help serve people. And now it will serve me and surround me with love and care during my journey. I leave with some hugs and head to the car.

Once in the car I break down and sob. Reality is setting in. This *is* *really* happening. I'm going to lose my breast and my life will be changed forever. I tell Bob to drive to the Solanus Casey Center for the healing service. I *need* to go there.

After leaving my intention and praying at Fr. Solanus' casket, I wait in line for a healing. The Brother giving the blessing happens to be someone I worked with on several fundraisers. He recognizes me and I tell him about my surgery. He touches my forehead with a relic of Fr. Solanus and prays. Bob is holding me; the brother is holding me. I feel the healing energy. *Peace.*

As I turn to leave, Bob stops me. He also wants a healing. This surprises me as he is very private about his faith. I'm reminded again this isn't just about me and my journey. He is dealing with cancer, too. I'm grateful to witness his healing. Holding him while he's being prayed over will be one of the most powerful moments in our marriage. A sharing of our faith. When I went into the church, I was weepy and sad, I leave feeling calm, at peace and empowered.

> *When life gives you more than you can stand—KNEEL.*
> —Gordon B. Hinkley

The Titty Wake
("Saying Goodbye to my Tata" Party)
May 31st—Later That Day

I've decided to have a goodbye party for my tata tonight. My friend Leslie dubbed it the "Titty Wake," which I think is so appropriate. My husband asked me if I was sure I wanted to do this the night before my surgery. I didn't hesitate; I absolutely wanted to have my lady friends surround me with their love and support. It's not the time to sit and wallow. We needed to celebrate my breast. This breast saved me. It is going to give me back my life. I'm grateful.

I wanted a night of celebration, not a night of sadness. I'm losing a breast; not losing my life. *Life changing*, not *life taking*. And I'm ready to get on with it.

There was food, wine, cake pops and cupcakes shaped like breasts. Everything was done up in pink. I had pink leis for everyone to wear. Of course, I got the ideas from Pinterest. Love Pinterest—it's like female fantasy football.

The night was perfect. We were celebrating my breast and the gift of life. I was surrounded by loving energy. I went to bed happy.

To my fellow goddesses who came to celebrate my breast, thank you for giving me a night filled with love and unconditional support. I love you all.

> *I get by with a little help from my friends.*
> —The Beatles

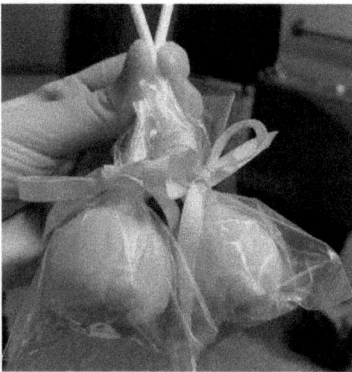
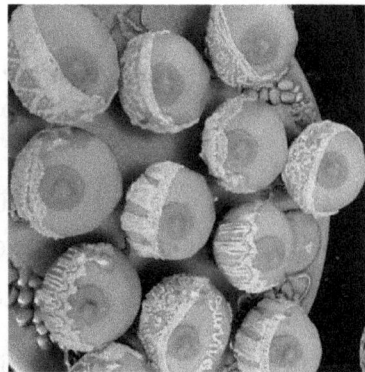

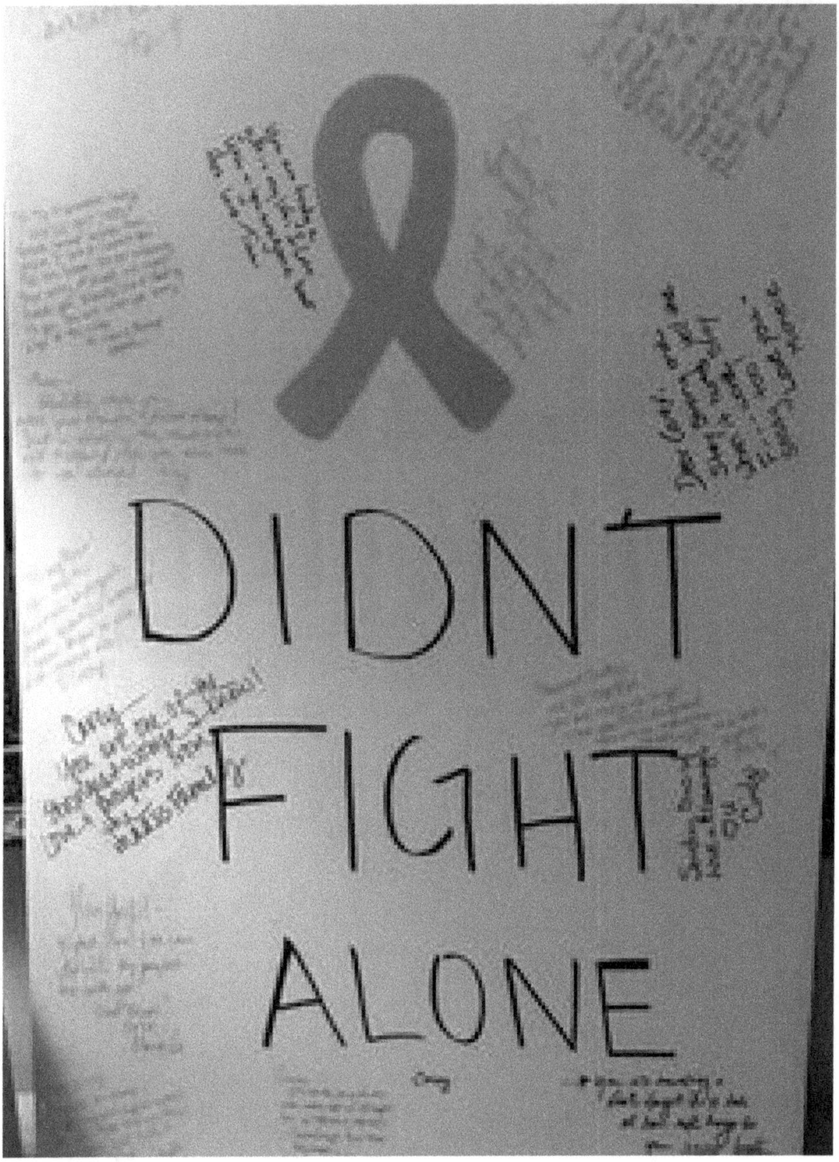
DIDN'T
FIGHT
ALONE

Mastectomy and Recovery

Can't Sleep
June 1st (Early Morning Hours)

It's 5 a.m. and I can't sleep. I've done some self-Reiki and attempted to meditate (as you can see that isn't happening). I've slept for three hours, and I feel compelled to write. Writing calms me.

It's dark out, I'm in my family room and I feel so lost and alone. You see, no one can do this for me. I have to do this by myself. It's the ultimate test of me. I'm heading into major surgery today. I will be put to sleep and wake up to one less breast. How will I look? How much will it hurt? Will I be able to manage the pain? The recovery? **Can I be brave?** One of my friends sent me a quote last night about being brave. *"Be brave. Remember that bravery is not the lack of fear but the ability to move forward in spite of fear."* There's no choice. I have to do this to live.

I choose life. Does that make me brave? I don't think so. Finding myself here today, leaving my house in an hour, I don't feel brave. I feel fear, sadness, apprehension, lonely and a little lost. But even feeling all that, I still feel gratitude. Gratitude cancer is only located in my left breast, gratitude the cancer is being removed today and gratitude for the journey I'm about to take. Because I know, as I learned last time, it will be filled with abundant love.

Cancer is like riding a roller coaster with peaks and valleys. Last week was a major roller-coaster ride. I met with the surgeon to find out my options. I went into the meeting with a mindset of double mastectomy and no other treatment and ended up with a plan of removal of one breast followed by chemo and radiation.

Not what I wanted. But even though it would be a battle, my prognosis for a longer life is great. I then had to have a bone and body scan to see if cancer had invaded any other parts of my body. I spent the entire weekend on pins and needles waiting for the results. I couldn't pull the trigger and tell the world until I knew. Good news on Tuesday. I was clear. Out of the valley.

Today, I will lose my breast. Once again, I'm in the dark. I have no idea how long the surgery will be. I have no idea what stage I'm in. I have no idea if it's in my lymph nodes (though Dr. Ruark thinks it's in at least one). I have no idea what treatment path I'm going to take. *I have no idea...* Once again, cancer is letting me know how unpredictable it is. It's showing me how I need to FLOW, that's all—just to go with the flow. I have no control—I HAVE NO CONTROL—so let it flow.

I will go into surgery, into the unknown. I will be in the unknown until test results come back. I will have the WAIT. The wait every cancer patient knows all too well. I will once again work hard at staying present, staying in the NOW, because that's what you do when you have cancer. You **wait** and you **hope,** and you **cope**.

I'm reflecting about my cancer right now. My first go-around, I was Stage 0/1a with a 97% cure rate. I had a clear mammogram last year. I was going into 6 years clear and now I'm at least Stage 2. How did this happen? I need to take my own advice this morning and realize it just is. Don't ask questions that have no answers and don't serve me. Let it go—**Flow**.

I'll take my shower in a few minutes and allow myself to cry. I'll hold my breast in gratitude and thank it for its service; for sacrificing itself so I can live. I will try to take my fear and **F**ocus the **E**nergy to **A**lter the **R**esult. I will get to know each and every person who helps me today and be thankful for their care. *Humor* will be present. I will open myself up to feel the love and strength being sent to me by so many family members and friends. *And I will be brave.*

> *When life gives you something that makes you feel afraid, that's when life gives you the chance to be brave.*
> —Lupytha Hermin

The Surgery—or Goodbye Cancer
June 1st

While heading to the hospital, I think about my ride for my first breast cancer surgery; how I was petrified and barely holding on to my sanity. Today, there is no fear, only peace. We listen to music, making sure it is upbeat and happy. Bob and Riley are lost in thought. I'm concentrating on the music; it helps my mindset.

We're just merging onto the expressway when my song—Earth, Wind & Fire's 'September'—comes on. I couldn't be happier! I'm dancing and jamming in the car. Life is great for me *right* at this moment. Today is a good and happy day. The cancer is being removed and will no longer be in my body. *It is* a day of gratitude.

We arrive early (that's a first). I'm wearing my pink lei in celebration of the day. Once checked in, an aide comes to walk me to my room. As soon as the doors swing open, she points to a scale. Really? Geez, I can't even get away from it today. Weight taken; I go to my room and get settled. I've brought some 'boob' cake pops to pass out to the doctors and nurses who will help me today. I'm in celebration mode.

I'm prepped for surgery. It takes two pokes to get the IV started. I'm hoping this isn't a bad omen. Radioactive dye will be injected into my breast so the doctor can see my lymph nodes "light up." The nurse warns me about the doctors who deal in this—"They're all weird and smell like moth balls." *Okay then, can't wait to meet mine.*

Lo and behold, in walks the same doctor I had 6 years ago. I say, "Hello, you're Slovak, right? You immigrated in the 80s." He's in shock that I remember his story from last time.

Still thinking about the mothball comment, I get him to tell me why he chose this profession. He likes to look at things and figure them out, he says. He's a quiet, serious man. I prefer the smiling, joking doctor, but in this case I'm fine with Dr. Serious. He's working with radioactive dye, after all. He carries it in a special black case that is locked.

Injections complete (there were two) and on to jiggling my breast. This is done to spread the dye around. I sit and 'jiggle' while I wait for my family to come back. My surgery was scheduled for 10 a.m., I'm told it won't happen now until 11:00.

I requested a Reiki session before my surgery. My family arrives at the same time as Sandy, the practitioner. I can hear my daughter crying outside the door. She's distraught and can't come in. My heart is breaking for her. I want her to know it's okay to cry and be sad, but we have to look at the big picture. I am coming away with my life. *IT IS A HAPPY DAY.*

I can hear Sandy soothe Riley before they come in. The Reiki treatment begins. Both Bob and Riley are on either side of me holding my hands. It's powerful receiving the energy going through my body. It leaves me feeling more at peace. We all seem calmer.

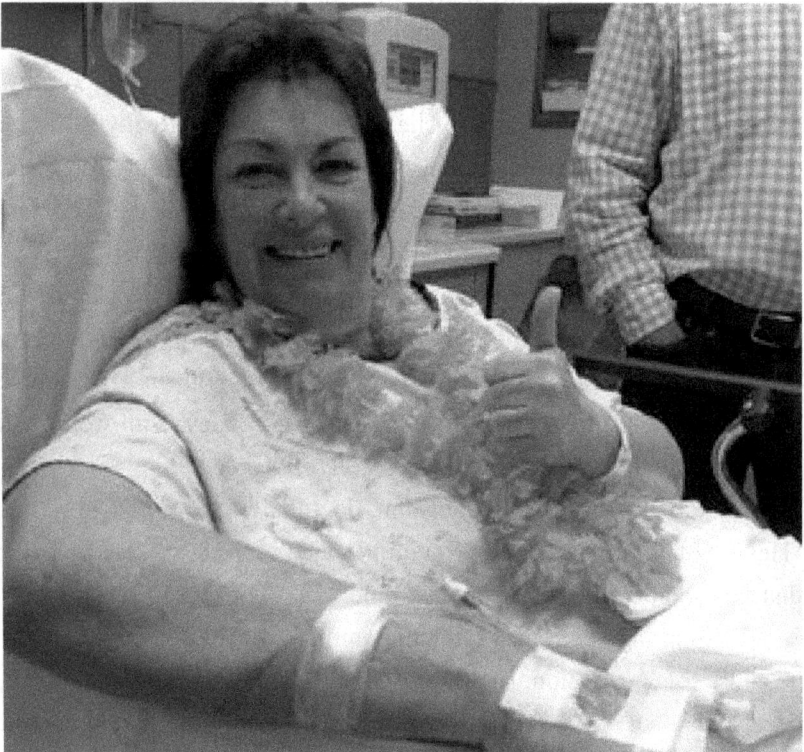

We sit, talk, and listen to music for the next two hours. I'm surrounded by Bob, Riley, my sister-in-law Renee, Auntie Dee and Uncle Jerry. The atmosphere is joyous. I hand out my 'boob' cake pops to all the personnel. The anesthesiologists are speechless. They smile and say this is a first. I've brought out some smiles today. In the midst of this crazy, sad/happy day, I smiled along with others.

Dr. Ruark comes in and I give her a cake pop. She smiles and sticks it in her pocket. She explains the surgery again. She tells me if I wake up and there are two drains in me that means the cancer has invaded my lymph nodes. I guess you know the first question I'll be asking when I wake up. She still anticipates the surgery will last around two hours.

They come in about 10:50 and say, *"Okay, it's time for the good stuff,"* and begin the injection into my IV. I don't remember anything after that (it really is good stuff). Renee told me later, I kissed everyone goodbye and then lifted my arms in the air saying, *"Whoop! Whoop! It's a happy day!"* as I was led out of the room and taken down the hall to surgery.

Bob stood at the door and wouldn't leave until he sees me turn the corner. He collapsed and sobbed after I was out of sight. When I hear about this later, I'm heartbroken for him. I think it's truly harder on my family watching me go through this. How sad and helpless they must feel. Cancer hasn't just rocked my world, but theirs also.

Time to Wake Up

I hear a man calling my name and begin to wake up. "We're taking you to your room, Carey." The surgery is done. As I'm wheeled to my room, my first thought is: How many drains? Once there, I ask my family: How many drains? Two. Two—that means the cancer was in my lymph nodes. *Dammit! Dammit! Dammit!*

I'm awake and in no real pain. I look down and my left side is flat. I don't want to look any further. I lay back and close my eyes. I will look later.

They tell me it went as expected. Dr. Ruark even did a little plastic surgery and tucked in the excess skin. She said she'd like all her patients to be as exuberant and positive as I am. I'm not trying to be anything but what I am. I can think of no other way to be during this. I must embrace this and hit it head-on, otherwise it will overtake me.

My mother and Denise come to see me. My mom just wants to give me a kiss. Isn't that wonderful? She needs to know I'm alright. While visiting, she keeps staring at me. I ask her what's wrong. She says nothing, I just can't get over how **good** you look. Who knew I could look good after surgery? ☺

I'm allowed liquids. They bring me chicken broth and ice chips. Bob, in his haste to help, spills the soup on me, not once but twice. I'm thinking about my decimation incident when I look at him and say, *"Hand me a straw."* The straw works perfect.

Everyone leaves and I finally sleep. Later, Bob comes back for the night. I've gotten out of bed, gone to the bathroom, and eaten all within six hours of surgery. Not too bad. I'm not feeling as awful as I thought I would.

Then again, I may have spoken too soon. In the middle of the night, feeling hot, nauseous, and turning green, I press the call button. The last thing I want to do is vomit. The kind and gentle aide puts cold compresses on my neck. I'm given anti-nausea medication and allowed to eat crackers and pudding. I begin to feel better. I'm coming back— *Whoo-hoo!*

Poor Bob is next to me sleeping on a chair bed snoring loudly. I ask them to shut the door so as not to disturb anyone else. I'm fine with his snoring. Seeing him sleeping so soundly, after the stress he went through today, makes me happy. He deserves a good night's rest.

As I lay listening to him snore, I think about this day. I went into the unknown this morning, underwent major surgery and will now begin healing. Even though I'm sad my breast is gone, and they found cancer in several lymph nodes, I'm relieved cancer is out of my body. I know my healing will take me through more peaks and valleys, and the fear of the unknown will come back at times. But tonight, laying in my hospital bed, the only emotion I feel is gratitude. Today *was* a great day!

> *Happiness is not always getting what you want all the time,*
> *it's about loving what you have and being grateful for it.*
> —Anonymous

The Morning After
June 2nd

While eating breakfast, I meet Dr. Ruark's physician's assistant. I've gotten conflicting information from the nurses and my doctor on the use of my left arm. My doctor tells me no movement until my drains are removed. Walking only to the bathroom and back. The nurses tell me to move my arm or risk frozen shoulder. The assistant confirms the doctor is correct. No computer, sitting still and doing nothing. OMG—this is worse than the surgery. *Yikes!* Will I be able to do this?

I'm allowed to leave after I eat lunch. (*Yay, one more hospital meal.*) Once home, I head straight for the new La-Z-Boy. This will be my spot for the next few weeks. Sitting, I think about my whirlwind 24 hours. I left my house with all my body intact. I've come home with one less breast. Though my body has been traumatized, it wasn't as awful as I imagined. I went into surgery smiling. I find myself smiling again, because I'm here and I no longer have cancer in my body. It's another good day. Let the healing begin!

> *It never hurts to keep looking for sunshine.*
> —Eeyore

The Shower
June 3rd

Bob knew I wasn't ready to see myself. I was having my first shower today. He told me to wait while he got things ready. Trust me, I wasn't going anywhere. I was moving *mighty* slow.

I noticed he had my sewing box (*not that I know how to sew, but I hear every household should have one*) along with some old T-shirts.

He had been working on something. He came back to help me out of my chair and take me back to our bathroom.

Once there, he turned me around, so I wasn't facing the mirror and helped remove my clothes. "Keep your eyes looking up," he says. I do. He has taken an old T-shirt and cut it in half and rigged the shoulder to cover me. This wonderful, incredible man made it, so I didn't have to look at myself.

He came in with me and helped me shower. I'm crying as I write this. I am so loved by him and am incredibly blessed. Done with the shower, he gently pats me dry. He dries my hair with me facing away from the mirror, making sure I don't look. In one of my most trying times, he makes me feel cherished. How did I get so lucky?

> *The single most extraordinary thing I've done in my life is fall in love with you.*
> —This is Us

Support from my Boys
June 4th

Riley can verbalize her feelings to me. I can talk with her and help her process. My boys are another story. Stoic and silent. They don't share how they feel. Whenever I ask questions, I always get the Cliff Notes version of an answer. I'm worried about them.

While I was in recovery, Riley showed me what Anthony posted on Facebook. It was a picture of me before surgery wearing my pink lei.

I'm speechless. Once I told him my diagnosis, he kept to himself. Working a lot, going to school, and when home he stayed in his room. I wasn't sure he was processing this well. When I read his post, it humbled me. He feels, he cares, and he loves. How lucky am I to have such a great kid? (Except for all those speeding tickets!)

Anthony Cornacchini with **Carey Ann Teets-cornacchini.**

Yesterday at 2:13 PM · Hazel Park · 👥

Prayers for my amazing Mother this afternoon everyone as she is in surgery. This is the second attempt cancer has tried to bring her down. Unfortunately cancer does not know my mother..nothing gets in her way not now not ever. She's a fighter! 🩶

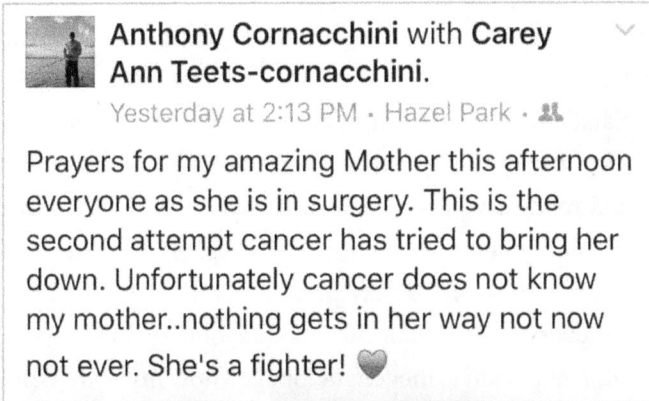

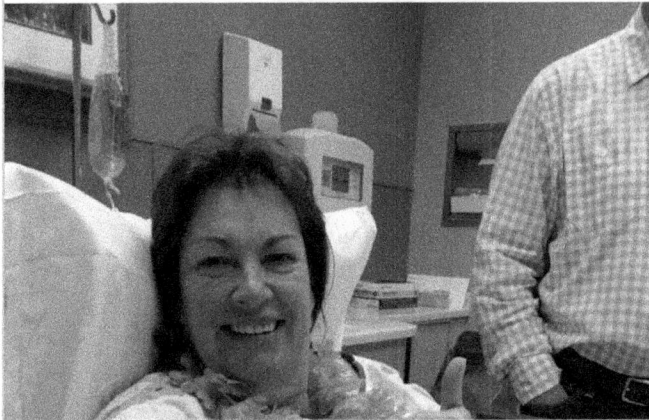

I tried to get my mastectomy delayed a week as Nick was having his bachelor party weekend the day after surgery. I wanted Bob to attend his son's party. Dr. Ruark stood firm. Surgery ASAP so I could begin treatment right away. No negotiation.

Nick wasn't sure he should go, maybe they should cancel the weekend. I was emphatic he attends. This was his time. I was just having surgery and would be fine. Cancer was not going to take away the joy of his wedding. We cannot let our lives revolve around this or let it take center stage. Thankfully, he decides to go.

Sitting in my ever-faithful lazy boy this afternoon; I feel myself entering a dark place. Here's the thing with cancer. Once discovered, it moves quickly. Mammogram, biopsy, mastectomy—Bing, bang, boom. It's been two weeks from diagnosis to surgery with multiple tests and doctor visits in between. I think my head finally caught up. I'm immensely sad and overwhelmed with it all. I begin to cry.

I call Natalie and talk for an hour. Her words help bring me back. *Balance.* Yes, I truly look at this in gratitude, but I can't always be sunshine and roses. I've *lost* a breast. I need to let myself mourn and grieve. This is traumatic, something life changing. Allow the grief.

Once again, remember to stay present. Don't think beyond today. With cancer, everyone has their own unique journey. I can't predict the type of treatment I'll have, the length, or even how my body will handle it; so, let it go. Stay in the now. *Breathe.*

I spend the day grieving. In the middle of my grief, Nick sends me a text. It's a picture of the entire group of guys at his bachelor party holding up a pink sign that says #savingteets. If I wasn't crying before, I'm sobbing now. Nick posted it on his Facebook and said:

> *Having a great weekend with all the boys. But can't help think about what's truly important. We all love you and are thinking about you, mom! #SavingTeets*

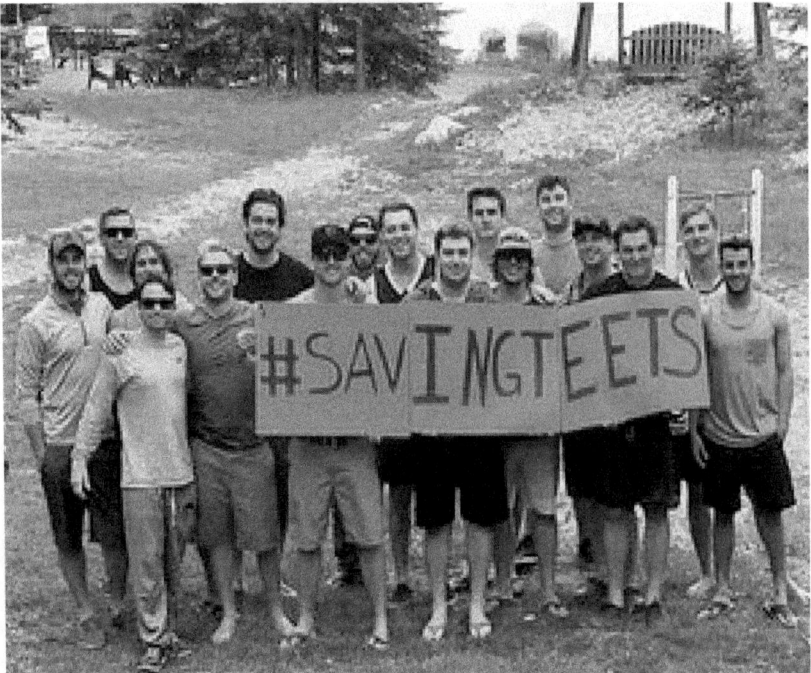

I'm told later they have spent over an hour trying to find pink poster board paper to make the sign. They took time from their bachelor party to think of me and support me. How did I get so blessed? My heart is bursting. The black cloud that was hovering over me just got lifted. It's amazing to me when I'm in the depth of a dark valley, something so loving and wonderful happens to bring me back to the peak. Once again, cancer has given me a gift. *Love*. I am loved.

> ***There is only one happiness in life, to love and be loved.***
> —George Sand

First Look
June 8th

Mentally, I knew what had happened. My breast was removed. Emotionally, I hadn't caught up yet. I was still processing. It wasn't as painful as I suspected. I was taking pain meds, but it was bearable. The drains weren't bothering me. I was slowly moving. But I still couldn't look at myself. I've looked down and could see my left side was flat, but I hadn't worked up the nerve to see my new body.

It's been a week since my surgery, and I have an appointment with my surgeon tomorrow. I need to see my chest before my appointment. My first look can't be in the doctor's office.

I'm getting ready to take my shower, my husband once again helping me. It was time. I take off the zip-up top I was wearing to hold in my tubes and face the mirror. I finally look.

I'm completely flat. There is nothing. When I say nothing, I *mean* nothing. There is a long scar covered with steri-strips and several other smaller scars. No nipple. **Nothing**. I think this is when it really hits me. I have breast cancer again and my body is scarred and mutilated. OMG—my husband has seen me like this all week and been nothing but loving. He's been telling me how beautiful I look. What a great job the surgeon has done.

I'm devastated and start sobbing. Crying for the breast I've lost; for everything I've been through, for the battle I've yet to fight. *I can't stop.* He holds me, while I cry, and tells me I'm beautiful. He reminds me this is temporary, that it will be fixed in the long run. He jokes, "Hey, look at the bright side. You'll get new perky breasts out of this." He's right. I need to look at the bright side and realize this is a means to an end. *That this is temporary.*

I look again, more clinically. There is little bruising, no swelling. I have no "chicken fat" on the side of my chest. I've heard from other women sometimes the extra skin is left for the plastic surgeon to fix. My doctor has done an excellent job.

After looking at myself clinically, I take another look. Obviously, my breast was hiding a *huge* secret. *My God, when did my stomach get that big? What the hell?* I just lost 50 pounds before diagnosis. I obviously need to step up my game!

I did it! First look over. Big girl panties on. I'm ready to heal and get to the next step.

> *Never be ashamed of a scar. It means you were*
> *stronger than whatever hurt you.*
> —Unknown

Pathology Report
June 8th—Later That Day

My friend Bev came to visit tonight. We worked together in the early 80s and have been great friends ever since. (Go Galligan's) Bev had Stage 2 lobular invasive breast cancer. She had a mastectomy and breast reconstruction. She got us to laugh when discussing the surgery. When she had it, her deductible had to be met for her to have a nipple put on her new breast. Her answer: "Why would I spend $1,200 for a raisin?" *Gotta love Bev!*

My doctor always gives me my test results as soon as she receives them. I get the call after Bev leaves. I had a tumor that was 12 cm., and four lymph nodes were positive for cancer. Waiting for good news here—and I receive it. All my margins are clear and I'm estrogen positive, which means I can take medication that will stave off cancer. Okay, I can deal with this. As part of my treatment, I will have chemo and radiation. Once again, something I didn't want to hear, but I need to look at those things as extra insurance to keep the Big "C" at bay.

> *Remember: things can be bad and getting better.*
> —Hans Rosling

Getting the Scoop
June 9th

We leave to see Dr. Ruark, I'm thrilled to get out of the house. You wouldn't think something so simple as riding in a car would excite me so much, but after sitting in a La-Z-Boy for a week 24/7, it's a treat!

An older woman with her two daughters come into the waiting room. We strike up a conversation. It's her second time on the Big "C" roller coaster also. This time it's gone to her other breast. We talk about our previous experience and how much we love Dr. Ruark. I'm in the presence of another club member. She understands me. She's been in the trenches. No one knows until they go through this what it's like. It's comforting knowing there are others like you, that you're not alone.

Dr. Ruark examines me and is happy at what she sees. She thought my skin would have been purple due to the previous radiation and she's pleasantly surprised. She tells us the same information as she did last night. I ask her what stage I'm in. Before surgery, she thought I'd be in Stage 2. Since they found cancer in a small fourth lymph node, it has put me barely into Stage 3. I'm not sure how I feel about that. I know we look at cancer in four stages, but I also know that there are different levels of stages. Last time, I was 0/1a. Now I'm 3b. I can't let myself get hung up on a number. My mantra comes into play, this is life-changing, not life-taking. CHANGING, NOT TAKING.

The clinical description

Stage IIIB (pT4b pN2a cMO) Grade 2 invasive lobular carcinoma of the ipsilateral left breast, ER/PR positive, HER-2 negative.

My description

The Big "C" is back again in a vengeance, the bastard!

She removes one tube. There is no pain. *Easy, breezy.* I still have one tube in, but it feels GREAT to have one removed. It's only been a week and one tube is removed. *Whoop! Whoop!*

While examining me, she sees I have a rash. This past week, I thought I had a heat rash. That would be a no. I'm allergic to the antibiotic. New script is ordered. *Thank God.* No more itching. Note to self: Call doctor next time and quit suffering silently.

Dr. Ruark asks about my children. I show her Anthony's Instagram post from the day of my surgery and Nick's picture with all the guys holding up the #savingteets sign. She starts to cry. She is so touched by them. She says: *"Don't show me anything else, I've got to see another patient and I can't go in crying."*

Bob is asking questions about the next steps. She has no answers, and I can see him getting frustrated. We need to realize treating cancer is compartmentalized. The surgeon does her job as does the oncologist and the radiologist. They all talk amongst themselves, but each is responsible for their own piece of the pie. Once again, we must learn to be patient and wait for the next steps. Dr. Ruark's office will make an appointment with the oncologist when my last drain is removed. *One day at a time, stay in the NOW. Breathe.*

As we're waiting for the elevator, I hug my husband and say, "This is a day of gratitude. I got out of the house, took a ride in our car, my body is cancer free, I have clear margins and I got one tube removed! *Whoop! Whoop!"*

> **Enjoy the little things, for one day you will look back and realize they were the big things.**
> —Robert Brault

My Dream
June 10th

I'm sick of watching television. I've watched all the old movies and shows I've recorded (50 episodes of "My Three Sons"—don't judge). Today, I leave the television off and spend my time listening to music and reading. I sleep off and on and dream. In my dream I'm at a walk for breast cancer. While walking, I look over and see both my grandfather's sitting together.

I run over to them, and my Grandpa Sloan says, *"Well, hello, Lover Dover"* (his nickname for me). I kiss him on his bald head, so happy to see him. I turn my head and there's my dad. I've never had my dad come to me in a dream before. He has tears coming down his face and says, *"I'm so sorry."* He reaches out and touches me and I actually feel his hand on my arm. I respond, *"It's okay, Dad, I'm going to be alright."* I wake up at peace and in my heart, I know I'm going to be just fine.

> **But the most important thing is, even if we're apart, I'll always be with you.**
> —A.A. Milne

Me and My Sidekick
June 11th

I've got a sidekick with me 24/7. It's my dog, Winston. We got him 16 years ago for our children. He's been mine ever since. I'm his mom and he loves me best. During my first journey with the Big C, he never left my side. I'd come home from surgeries or treatment, and he couldn't get on my lap fast enough.

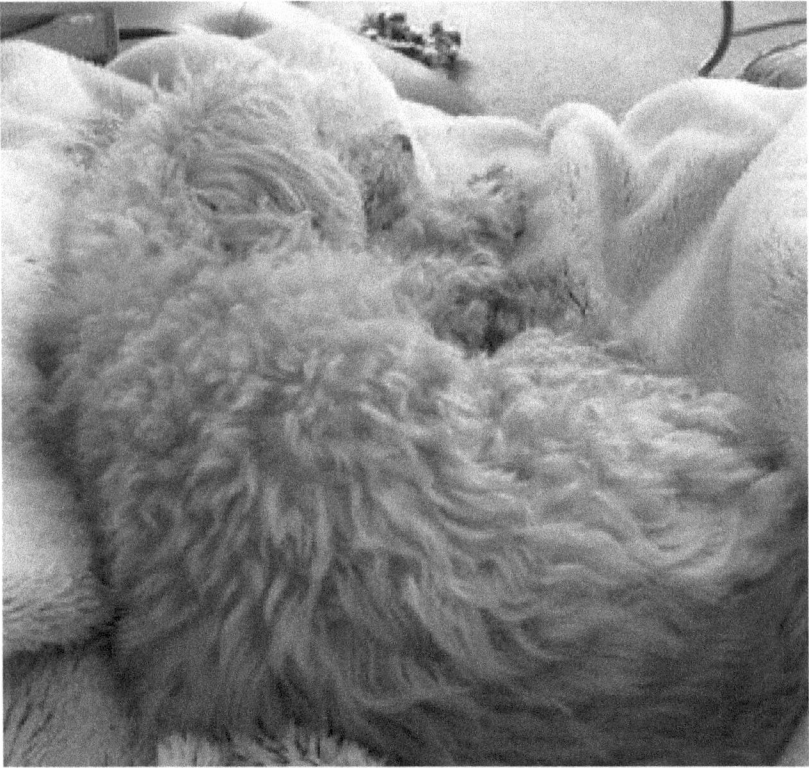

He senses I have cancer. I know it and feel it. He gets frantic when he can't be with me. He paces and cries. He can't really jump up on couches and chairs anymore, so he must be lifted. Once he's in my lap, he always sighs with contentment. And guess what? I do too.

Winston's 16 now. He sleeps longer and moves slower. He has horrendous breath—LOL. Anthony laments we have the old smelly dog. We've been told we can't clean his teeth as he has a slow beating heart, and the anesthetic will most likely kill him. So smelly teeth it is.

I've resorted to feeding him human food. He gets ground sirloin, chicken or ground ham always accompanied by shredded cheese, of course. Spoiled, yes, but with all the energy and unconditional love he's given us over the years, he deserves it.

When I received my diagnosis, I said to him, "You're 16 and nearing the end of your time here, but I need you to hold on a little bit longer for me." (*Yes, I discuss things with him all the time—great listener, no backtalk.*) I know it's selfish, but I'm not ready to let him go. He's an integral part of my journey. He gives me such great energy and love and I can't imagine going through it without him. From the bottom of my heart, thank you, Winston, for being my shadow.

> **I think dogs are amazing creatures; they give unconditional love. For me they are the role model for being alive.**
> —Gilda Radner

Progress
June 13th

If all looks well; I will have my second drain removed today. I'm cautiously optimistic. Once in the room, Theresa begins to exam my drain, its output and color. There was nothing as I've emptied 3 cm of tan colored fluid before I came. I'm excited that there's very little liquid now. Mentally, I'm keeping my fingers crossed.

Before we deal with my remaining drain, she discusses my port. She shows me a port and explains how it will be surgically inserted along with possible side effects. (Yep, not going there.) We discuss possible dates. It may happen as early as next week, with chemo beginning the following week. *Say what? I haven't even seen the oncologist yet.* Once again, this is moving way too quickly for me.

I was hoping for some downtime to go away for a long weekend. I want to regroup before I begin the next part of my journey. She's not sure if it will happen. *Keeping my fingers crossed.*

Theresa discusses hair loss. She tells me about a free class offered to cancer patients on how to do makeup, hair/wig tips, etc. I will be attending; Lord knows I need all the help I can get.

She leaves the room and I turn to Bob and choke up. He asks what's wrong. I respond, *"Oh, just the usual, reality hitting me."* It comes in waves. I'll find I'm going about my day, and something will hit me and even at times steal my breath away when I think about this journey. I then work hard to bring myself back to the present and realize I'm just one of many who has had to take this path. It's a path I'm taking because I choose life. It's really that simple. I allow myself to take in the moment whether it be fear or sadness, but I don't allow it to consume me. I acknowledge it but move on to peace.

Theresa comes back in the room and does an ultrasound on my neck. She's checking veins for my port. It will be inserted into my right side, not my left where the cancer is located. Bob asks why. The right side works better for the flow. Interesting. Good veins found. Now on to the last drain. She decides my drain can be removed.

I let her know I felt no pain when Dr. Ruark removed the last drain, so the pressure is on. "Oh great," she says, "Dr. Ruark probably removed the shorter one," which she did. I feel a slight pull and it's out. *Whoop! Whoop! Freedom!* She still wants me to take it easy for the day and gives me exercises to help in raising my arm.

Theresa asks if anyone has shown me a breast prosthetic. Ugh, that would be no. She explains I will receive a script and be fitted for a prosthetic and a mastectomy bra. *Great, someone else will be touching me there.* I'll be honest: My breasts are heavy. I'm sure I lost 5 pounds when my breast was removed. I'm hoping for a 'light' prosthetic. She brings one in and hands it to me. It's squishy and is just as heavy as my real breast. Really? Can't I catch a little break? I turn to my husband and say, "When I replace these babies, I'm getting size B."

Drain out; information given. On the way out, I get my appointment with the oncologist. It's set for tomorrow at 5:30. Another hurdle *down*.

> *A great accomplishment shouldn't be the end of the road, just a starting point for the next leap forward.*
> —Harvey McKay

Prepping for Treatment

Oncology 101
June 14th

D r. Hanna has squeezed us in as his last appointment of the day. I'm nervous. I **really** don't want to have chemotherapy. Out of all my treatments for the Big "C", chemo is the one I'm dreading. My nerves are getting the best of me. On the ride there, I meditate. Taking in slow breaths, in and out, mentally saying to myself, "Calm in, fear out." Breathing, really taking conscious breaths, helps.

Once in the examination room I'm given pages and pages of paperwork to fill out. I notice most of the questions are the same questions I seem to have to answer for every doctor I see. I need to make a copy and just bring it with me wherever I go.

Prior to this visit, I've thought about my treatment. So many questions popping into my head. *What will the duration be? Will I be sick? Will it hurt?* I'm obsessed about the unknown. Every time I think about it, I have to bring myself back. It doesn't serve me. Stay present. *Will you ever learn Carey?*

Dr. Hanna comes in. He's a gentle, quiet, kind man. I like him immediately. He delves right into my family history and the fact my mother and aunt had breast cancer. I let him know I've had the genetic testing, and it wasn't hereditary. We go over my last bout with the Big "C," what stage I was in, what type of treatment, etc. He asks if I had regular mammograms. Yes, every four months for the first two years, followed by every six months for a year, then once a year after that.

We move on to my current cancer. He reiterates its invasive lobular cancer and is slow growing, which is good. I ask if this cancer has grown within a year since my last mammogram was clear. He says, maybe longer. Then he drops the bomb: **Mammograms don't usually pick up invasive lobular cancer**. Seriously? All the money and research and we don't have a conclusive test for invasive lobular cancer? *Well, that settles it, for sure, the other tata is going.*

My body and bone scans are clear, another plus. Since it's Stage 3, I need to have chemo and radiation. He emphasizes I will be on an estrogen blocker for at least 10 years, and how this treatment is more important than chemo.

I took tamoxifen during my last journey; the side effects were awful. I didn't complete the five years. I opted out after a lengthy discussion with my previous oncologist. (I was told I had a 97% cure rate and was Stage 0/1a.) We discuss the side effects. He says since I'm postmenopausal, they should be easier. Either way, I tell him, I will take it. (Not that I'm happy about it.)

When we're through with my history, he examines me and says I'm healing well. He asks if I work. I tell him I am a Reiki practitioner here in the infusion center. Full circle, I tell him. Examination complete. Clothes back on, ready to hear the plan.

Dr. Hanna begins to tell us the chemo regimen. The chemo is given to ensure any rogue cells which have gone elsewhere will be killed off. *I'm all for that.*

The most intense chemo, A/C (Adriamycin/Cyclophosphamide), will be given first. There will be four rounds, once every two weeks for eight weeks. Once this is complete, I will then be given another form of chemo—Taxol (a less intense treatment)—once a week for 20 weeks, so twenty-eight weeks in total. Well, I guess I know what I'll be doing for the next *seven* months.

Dr. Hanna wants me to heal for a few more weeks before we begin. I need to get a heart echo and the port inserted prior to treatment. He's thinking I'll start either the first or second week of July. That's just a month before Nick's wedding (August 19th) which is my biggest concern. I want as much energy as possible. He assures me they will work around it. I'm relieved.

"Can I have my chemo Wednesdays in Troy?" I ask. He asks why. "That's day I volunteer. I feel at home there and know I will be well taken care of. These ladies are my peeps." He agreed with a smile.

"What's the timeframe for reconstructive surgery?" We were thinking early next year. *Nope.* He says after I have radiation, I will have to wait at least six months for my skin to heal. A year. I will be dealing with this for 12 to 18 months minimum. Much longer than the 60 days I had with my last dance with the Big "C".

"What about exercising?" I do water aerobics four days a week. He thinks it's an excellent idea. *Whoop! Whoop!* I'm coming back to the pool, ladies. Some normalcy.

I want to know when I'll lose my hair. Probably after the second treatment, he says. (Better order my wig) Bob asks when it will come back. Not until I'm done with chemo. *Seven months without hair, oh well, easier to get ready.*

"When will the chemo side effects hit me?" He replied, "Usually it's between four and five days after the infusion." This is when my white cell count goes down and I will feel exhausted. Anti-nausea medication will be given at the same time as the chemo to offset the nausea. Okay, I'm looking for the silver lining here—and I've found it. Nauseous and no appetite. Losing some weight before the wedding. That's a *positive*.

Throughout our discussion, Dr. Hanna stops at times and just looks at me. I think he's assessing how I'm digesting this. He's trying to be very gentle. I keep smiling at him, I almost want to reassure *him*. Listen, I tell him, everyone has something, everyone has a story, this is just mine. The mantra is life changing, not life taking. He smiles at that. He says he will be seeing a lot of me during this process. I tell him I'm glad. He gets up to shake my hand and looks me in the eye and says, "I know you're going to handle this just fine." And you know what? I am.

On the way home, my husband looks at me and says, *"We can do this."* (I love when he says, "we.") *"We will just create a new normal."* He's so right. Isn't he fantastic?

I'm not going to say I'm not fearful of chemo, because I am. I have no idea how my body is going to respond to the chemicals being put into it, but it is a necessary 'evil' to make me whole. I will think of it as my helper in my healing journey.

I've stated many times about this being a battle. I don't want the pressure of "battling" or being referred to as brave. Why add more negative energy to it? I'm just one of millions who are navigating their way through life with cancer. I'm *healing*, that's all. Cancer is just another part of my life journey.

When you receive the diagnosis, you understand what's truly important, *Love*. Rather simple but profound. Love for the healing I will receive, for all the lessons and gifts it will give me, and for all the people who will help me during my journey. And most importantly for the love and care I give to myself. All the surgery, chemo, and radiation are just a part of me loving myself for choosing this path.

I've decided to look at the next phase as my new job—*having chemo to help me heal.* I will go to my treatments and follow and execute everything which is told to me. I will manifest a positive, loving experience because: A mastectomy, chemo, radiation, and an estrogen blocker will give me a longer life. I'm going to rock this 'job.'

> *Attitude is a little thing that makes a big difference.*
> —Winston Churchill

Barcelona Here She Comes
June 19th

Today's the day. Riley flies to Barcelona to begin her study abroad program. Her flight leaves at 11 a.m. I get up early and lay with her; holding her with the dog in between us. Where else would Winston be? She silently starts to cry. She doesn't know it, but I do, too. I know this is hard for her. And it's hard for me to see her this way.

Anyone would naturally be apprehensive doing an internship in a different country but adding the extra stress of a mom going through cancer is difficult. I'm thankful she is going with one of her best friends. They will be living together in an apartment. However, she and her friend have been placed in different internships, so she'll be navigating on her own. Big steps, a huge milestone for Riley. She's conflicted about leaving right now; she wants to stay and help take care of me.

One of Riley's biggest fears is the changes she'll see when she comes back. I talk honestly about it. My hair will be gone. I'll probably shave it before it falls out. She asks me why. Why not just cut it really short? My response: *I want to be in control. I don't want to pull my hair out in clumps.* She understands. She tells me to get several wigs and switch it up. I may just do that. I'll ask Bob if he's ever wanted to be with a blonde or a redhead.

There will be times when she calls, I'll be exhausted. I let her know not to panic over it, this is just my body responding to the chemo. I will get my energy back. All this is temporary. A *necessary* temporary situation. Remember the mantra, "Life changing, not life taking." We talk about how in life, the most challenging circumstances always bring out the most growth. (And this is certainly making us grow.)

I remind her she's realizing one of her dreams today; how she made it happen through her hard work. Yes, it will be scary to navigate the first few weeks. She will get homesick, but she must remember to embrace the adventure.

I let her know she's a little like me right now, facing the unknown. I could let fear win and crawl into myself, or I can embrace it and all the gifts it will give me. She can decide what type of journey she'll have. We talk a bit longer and hold each other, giving each other comfort. Of course, with Winston right there getting some love. We eventually close the suitcase and head to the airport.

Once there, we meet up with Kirsten. She will be the yin to Riley's yang. A great combination. We meet her parents and it's interesting to see both dads have the same worries. Bob ends with "And no Latin lovers, girls."

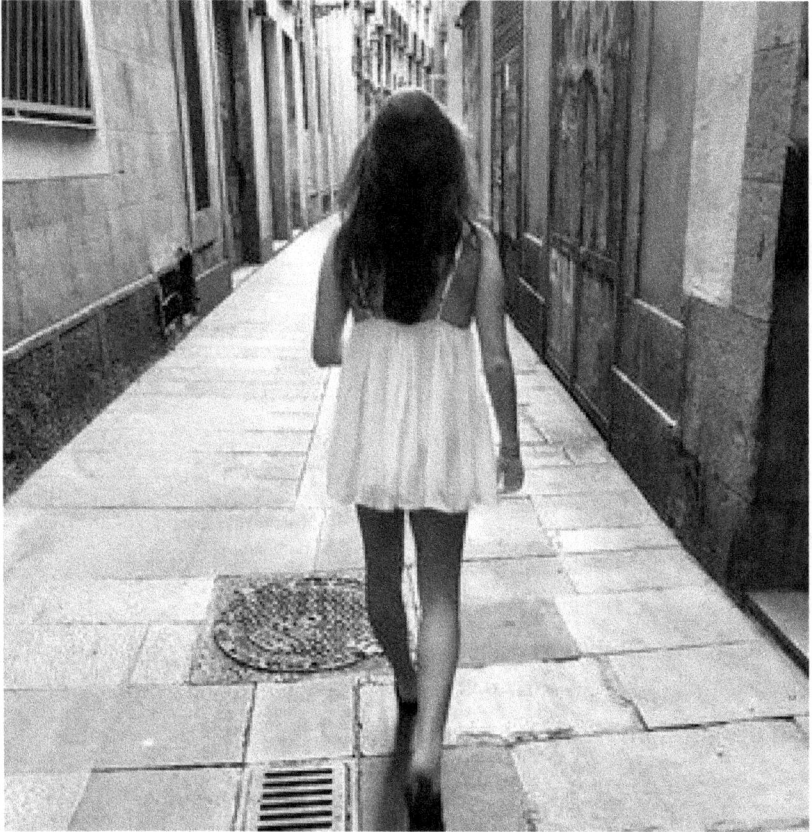

It's time to say goodbye. Riley and I hug, and tears start to flow. Happy and sad at the same time. We're both embarking on journeys into the unknown. She to explore the world and expand her horizons. Me to embrace the next phase of my cancer journey. I look into her eyes and say, "You're going to be just fine, Riley," and she responds, "And so are you, Mom."

> *Attitude is the difference between an ordeal and an adventure.*
> —Bob Bitchin

Information Overload! (Busy, Busy, Busy)
June 20th

I have several appointments today. A heart echo, a visit to check on the healing of my mastectomy and then an appointment with the oncology nurse to discuss my chemo regimen.

You've got to have heart . . .

Dr. Hanna has ordered a heart echo. There is a slight chance the chemo can damage my heart (*what a side effect!*) Before I begin treatment, they want to make sure my heart is fine. Getting all the tests done was a little unnerving. My entire body was being looked over. I already had cancer. I really don't want to find anything else.

My ever-present husband takes me to the appointment since I still can't drive. (*Talk about feeling trapped*) I'm the only one there and get in immediately. I meet Kristen, who will be doing the procedure. She's very kind, married, has three kids (including two-year-old twins) and has been doing this for several years. Yep, I did it again. I need to bond with people treating me.

She asks me if I still have drains. I tell her no and she tells me about a woman who came in and still had four drains. Four drains! Poor thing. I had two and was miserable, but four? Once again, I'm reminded how lucky I am.

I'm to strip from the waist up (*no surprise there*) and put on a hospital gown. I'm still very sore and lifting my arms is difficult. After a little maneuvering, I'm ready to go.

Kristen has me lay on my left side. *Yikes*, that's where the mastectomy was done. I gingerly lay down. She applies warm gel and begins. The process takes all of five minutes and I'm done. It takes me longer to put my clothes back on then the entire procedure.

Check-in

After my heart echo, we head to Dr. Ruark's office. I meet with Theresa. She checks my scarred area and feels my healing is progressing nicely. Second appointment done!

We head to lunch in the cafeteria. We finish early so I decide to head up to the integrative medicine office to see my friends and make an appointment with the naturopath oncologist to discuss additional help for my journey.

I'm greeted with warm smiles and hugs. It's like coming home. My appointment with Dr. Walker is set for Tuesday, June 27. One more step in the process. I want the marriage of the two factions, Western and integrative medicine, for treatment. Knowledge is power.

Last appointment *(or information overload)*

We head to Dr. Hanna's office and meet Donna. She will be my oncology nurse during chemo. We discuss the phases of my chemo treatment. She repeats some of the information Dr. Hanna gave to us, but in more detail.

I will receive Adriamycin/Cyclophosphamide (A/C) chemo first. (From now on I will be writing it as A/C.) It will be the strongest of the treatments. She repeats the schedule that Dr. Hanna told me. I've heard from friends who have had this refer to it as the Red Devil. Makes you stop and pause, doesn't it?

The side effects of the A/C are more intense than the Taxol. Nausea, extreme fatigue, possibility of heart palpitations, achy bones. Usually, people feel the side effects three to five days after the infusion. I will be fatigued because my white cells drop. They will build back up and I will feel around 85% to 95% after two weeks. Hence the reason for the two-week cycle.

I will have to receive Neulasta the day after my treatment. It helps reduce the risk of infection. I have a choice of either going to the hospital the next day or wearing a patch for 27 hours, which will provide my injection. I haven't made my decision yet.

I once again ask when I will lose my hair. I've already asked the doctor, so why ask the nurse? I think about it later and I guess I was hoping for a different answer. She tells me usually between the first and second treatment. There is a 50/50 chance I'll lose my eyelashes and eyebrows. Now *that* really upsets me. I'm ready to lose my hair, but losing my eyebrows? That's another story.

The entire infusion process will take about three hours. First, I will be given anti-nausea medication via IV, followed by Benadryl, then a steroid. Then Adriamycin is administered by the nurse; followed by an IV drip of the Cyclophosphamide. She tells me it will immediately change the color of my urine to red, so I won't be alarmed. My first treatment will take four to five hours as they will have me stay to make sure I'm tolerating it.

Donna gives me three prescriptions. Two are for anti-nausea medication. I am to take these religiously. Like taking pain meds—stay on top of it. If the first script is not working, take the second right away. The goal is to keep it tolerable. Eat small meals throughout the day. She tells me not to worry about diet. Eat what tastes good. There will be a time where I won't have taste buds. This will be temporary. *Now there's a positive, eat anything I want.*

The last prescription is for lidocaine, a numbing cream. I'm to slather it on my port area and cover it with cling wrap an hour before I go to the hospital. This will numb the area, so I won't feel the tube going in the port. My first thought when I hear this is: how big is the tube? Since it sounds like it's painful, bring on the lidocaine.

I will see my oncologist after my first treatment to assess how my body is handling the chemo. Once I've completed the A/C portion of the treatment, I will move on to Taxol.

She tells me this will be less taxing. Most patients handle this just fine with minimal side effects. I will have this once a week for 12 weeks. I stop and look at her. Twelve weeks? Not twenty? I misheard Dr. Hanna. I thought I had to have Taxol for 20 weeks with a total of

28 weeks of treatment. It's a total of 20 weeks of chemo treatment. *Life just got brighter.*

There are side effects which can occur after Week 5. There may be bone and joint pain and numbness in my fingers and toes. She emphasizes I need not suffer in silence. It's imperative to let them know if I have a low-grade fever, or vomiting, any achy joints, etc. There are things to help. I will need to stay hydrated. She stresses to drink a minimum of two liters of water per day. Ginger is my friend; hard candies, Tums, Rolaids, and saltines will help.

We leave on information overload. While digesting this, we look at each other, hug and say, "*This is doable. We can do this.*" We're navigating this journey together and I couldn't be happier I have him by my side.

I get my heart echo results later. My heart is just fine. Let's see, heart echo fine—check. Body scan clear—check. Bone scan clear—check. Chest X-ray clear—check. Blood work fine—check. And then—breast cancer in my left breast. Healthy as a horse except for a little breast cancer. LOL

> *Together we can get through this struggle called life.*
> —Unknown

A Port in Any Storm
June 20th

As I'm checking in at the hospital, one of the ladies says, "Were you here two weeks ago wearing a pink lei?" "Yep, that was me," I answer. She laughs and responds, "I remember you." I hope it was a good impression. 😊

In my presurgical room to get prepped, I'm apprehensive as it took two pokes to set up my IV the last time and I had a huge bruise that lasted a few weeks. This time, as I'm giving my information to the nurse, Theresa, aide, Anna, is attempting to put in my IV. Attempting would be the keyword here. I tend to talk while that's going on. Distraction helps. They first inject you with lidocaine to numb the area (which should tell you there is a large needle to follow). There's a burning sensation that follows the injection, but trust me, it's worth it.

While discussing my surgical history with the nurse, I tell them about bringing the boob cake pops to celebrate my last surgery. They laugh and say, "You're the one! We're still talking about those cake pops!" Glad I brought some smiles to people that day.

Meanwhile, Anna makes her first attempt. Yep, you heard me, first attempt. Stinging sensation complete, needle goes in, and it doesn't thread. Okay then, let's try again. This time she tries a vein on top of my hand. Stinging sensation complete, needle goes in and once again it doesn't thread (whatever that means). I'm not a happy camper right now. Anna turns to the nurse and says, I'll go get a nurse anesthetist. Oh boy, this is not sounding good. Anna leaves. Theresa takes over.

As Theresa is looking over my veins (which, honestly, is truly an uncomfortable feeling, like spinning the roulette wheel), in walks Tom. I ask, "Who are you?" He laughs and says, "I like that you asked me that." Theresa does poke three on the side of my hand, and it works. Tom, who came to the rescue, wasn't needed. The three of us discuss the pros and cons of nurse practitioners versus physician's assistant. What I got out of this: Nurse practitioners have more autonomy and next time around I'll only let the nurse set up my IV.

Bob comes in and we wait. I turn on Pandora and listen to music and listen to a little Earth, Wind & Fire. I'm grooving. Dr. Ruark comes in and says she'll be with me in a few minutes. Something must have come up because she arrives a half an hour later.

She's examining my mastectomy site and asks when I begin chemo. I tell her July 12th. She is not a happy camper. She explains how she likes things to progress quickly. Studies have shown that with Stage 3 cancer, quick treatment helps ensure no reoccurrence. She wants me to call my oncologist and start a week earlier. I tell her we are working around the wedding, so I'll have energy. Her response? They'll just be happy you're there.

My immediate response is anger. I value her opinion. I literally trust her with my life and for the first time I don't agree with her. I've listened to her throughout this process, and she has always helped me understand the reasons behind decisions, I'm just so focused on the wedding, I don't want to begin chemo earlier.

This has just thrown me into a tailspin. She leaves and I start to get worked up. Bring it back, Carey. Not a good way to go into surgery. I work hard at letting it go. I know deep down, she only has my best interests at heart, and I'm not mad at her, I'm upset about the timing. My focus is to feel the best I can at Nick's wedding. I decide I'll worry later, like Scarlett O'Hara, I'll think about it tomorrow.

I'm having twilight sleep this time as the surgery will last only 50 minutes. I'm given a sedative, kiss my husband and off I go. This time I'm awake when I get to the operating room and move myself onto the table. In previous surgeries I was already out when wheeled into the room, which means I had to be lifted on the table. Yikes! That is not a good visual.

Surgery complete. I'm in recovery and not too sore. I can't go home until I've eaten. I have some graham crackers and cranberry juice, get the okay and then leave. Note to self: Bringing one's truck to drive home after surgery is not a great idea. It's never good to climb after surgery. Will we ever learn?

When home I promptly fall asleep. Recovery, once again, begins. I am sore, and my body knows it has a port. That night, I sleep in the La-Z-Boy. It keeps me upright and cocooned. Of course, after sleeping all day, I wake up at 2 a.m. and am not able to go back to sleep. I watch TV, read, listen to music, and *think*.

It's weird I have this in my body. I feel it when I move, particularly in my neck. Will it feel like this the entire time? Will my body adjust to it? I'm told this will make the infusion easier on me. I think about my port and what it means. It is my lifeline of sorts. Its job is to administer my chemo, the 'potion' to help me heal and live a longer life. It has a significant role in my journey. And, even though I'm uncomfortable, I'm grateful for it.

> *Gratitude is an art of painting an*
> *adversity into a lovely picture.*
> —Kak Shri

Blindsided
June 21st

It's the day after the surgery and I'm on the phone with someone. While discussing my port, I tell her I had a day of anger yesterday. Anger about the timing of my chemo. Frustration at being poked and prodded and being sore but my mindset was better today. Her response: *You need stop the façade of acting so positive. It's so fake.* I'm crushed; she has wounded me. My response: "But, I *am* positive. Yes, I have bad days, but I choose not to stay there."

Off the phone, I feel sad, hurt, and angry. Navigating cancer is hard, both mentally and physically. I work every day at staying present and keeping my mind positive. I'm the glass is half-full kind of gal and see humor in just about everything. I refuse to let cancer take that away and to have someone say something so callous crushes me. Someone who has never experienced cancer felt empowered to tell me how to handle it. I'm reeling.

After stewing for a while, I realize I let someone's words bring me down. I gave away *my* power to someone who has *no* empathy. I've learned a valuable lesson here. Never again allow someone's cruel words to affect my inner peace. Negativity is not welcome in my life.

> *Life is too short to let someone make you*
> *miserable. Remember someone can only make you*
> *unhappy if you give them the power to do so.*
> —Unknown

Long Week
June 23rd

I find I'm uncomfortable most of the week. I'm unable to go to Traverse City for my future daughter-in-law's bachelorette weekend because I can't sleep in a bed. I'm angry. Cancer is once again affecting my life. *I hate this!*

It takes me a few days to get out of my funk, working hard at bringing myself into the light. I realize all of this is just a part of my journey; this is the bad that comes with the good. Yes, I'm sore and uncomfortable, but it's the by-product to help me live. That's all. This is all *temporary*. A means to an end. Every day when you wake up, you have a choice. You can choose to be negative or positive. I choose positive. It's as simple as that.

> *Life is a choice that you make every day to change and empower yourself. Choose to be true, to be positive and to be happy. NO MATTER WHAT.*
> —Venkat Desireddy

It Pays to Have Friends in High Places
June 24th

When I was diagnosed, I knew I wanted to talk with my friend, Maureen. We met when our sons attended preschool together, almost 30 years ago. We've both been on a journey of holistic healing. She transformed her career from ER doctor to head of Integrative Medicine. Me, becoming a Reiki practitioner. Okay, her journey was harder and touches many more lives, but I'm trying.

Knowing I wanted to use the services of Integrative Medicine, she was the perfect person to speak with. Her husband, Joe is an oncologist and could give me a second opinion regarding my treatment. Speaking with both together—double bonus!

I wanted Joe's opinion regarding the timing of my chemo treatments. Joe is amazing. He talks for over an hour, explaining everything to us. He begins going over my scans—all clear except for a touch of arthritis in my back. Explaining what type of cancer I have, it's good news. Estrogen positive and high success in cure rates.

Joe breaks down the entire diagnosis, so we understand. I notice something during this. Normally, I'm the one who is taking notes during these types of visits. This time it was Bob asking all the questions, writing down things. I was quiet. When thinking about it later, I realized I was uncomfortable talking about me. Hearing the success of treatments along with the cure rate makes me think about my mortality. Will I be on the upside of success, or will I be the percentage that doesn't succeed? Once again, I'm going places I don't need to go. *God, cancer is such a mind game!*

I explain to Joe, Dr. Ruark's concerns about beginning my chemo a week later than she wants. He tells me it's fine to begin on the date scheduled. *Whoo hoo!* That was worth the visit alone.

Joe reminds me to stay present. Reiterating what Natalie has told me. "Don't think about the length of treatment," he says. It could overwhelm me. Stay in the now, take each day as it comes.

Maureen speaks about Integrative Medicine and how it can work in conjunction with traditional medicine. Acupuncture to help with nausea and neuropathy. Herbs and vitamins to help with side effects. Massage and, of course, Reiki. She reiterates that Dr. Walker, who is a naturopath oncologist, will help me navigate my journey.

We leave feeling blessed to have these people in our lives. They've taken time to help us understand my diagnosis and treatment and given us something so rare in the Big "C" journey—peace. Once again, cancer has given me an amazing gift, wonderful friends who care.

> *Friendship is another word for love.*
> —Unknown

Another Reality Check
June 25th

I had just run out of shampoo and was shopping in TJ Maxx. They had Nioxin in a gigantic bottle at a great price. *Happy dance.* Love getting those deals. I gleefully put it in my cart.

Later, as I'm in line to check out, I have an epiphany. I'm not going to have hair within a month and will not likely have any for at least a year. Why am I buying this huge bottle of shampoo?

I take it out of my cart and walk back to the hair products area. I stand and look at the wall. Staring at the curling irons, hair dryers and brushes. I won't be needing these soon. I get a little melancholy realizing I'm not going to shampoo my hair for a very long time because I won't have hair to wash. Reality is sinking in. I end up going next door to Ulta and buy a travel-size shampoo.

> *Reality hurts when you fight it. It makes you strong when you accept it.*
> —Maxime Lagace

Shopping for My Wig
(AKA the Cranial Prosthetic)
June 26th

Since I'm going to lose my hair; I've looked at all my options for when I do. Hats, scarves, wigs, or au natural. I've decided to purchase a wig. I think a wig will help me feel normal.

I've made an appointment at Advance Hair Solutions. I asked my beautician and friend, Debbie, if she would shave my head when the time comes, and she readily agrees. She offers to accompany me wig shopping. I gladly take her up on her offer.

Bob and I arrive and it's surreal. There are rooms filled with mannequin heads with wigs. Faceless, just staring at you. It's kind of creepy. We meet Pamela, who is very kind. She explains about the wigs, hair loss, eyebrow loss, etc. I know I'm going to lose my hair, but losing my eyebrows bothers me. She tells me about a product called EES which helps prevent loss. It's a liquid which is to be applied twice a day. If it might save my eyebrows, I'm in. It's expensive: $135 for two ounces. I don't care. Sign me up.

Debbie arrives and we begin. I tell Pamela I want real hair. I don't want people to be able to tell I'm wearing a wig. (*Just had a revelation writing this: All my family and friends know I'm going through chemo, right? So, when I have my wig on, they're going to know it's a wig*).

Pricing is hefty, from $1,200 to $3,500. I try on a few. They're just not doing it for me. I don't like the way I look. And me as a blonde—*scary*! Then Pamela drops a bomb on me: If I have real hair, I will have to style it every day. Okay, those who know me know this is something I'm terrible at. When I had a daughter after having two boys, one of my first thoughts was OMG I have to do girl hair? I will not only lose my hair, but then wear a wig that needs to be styled every day. So not fair. I'm beginning to think a synthetic wig is my best option.

Pamela convinces me to try some synthetic wigs. She tells me they've come a long way, and they look and feel like real hair. And bonus: *They're styled*. There is a silver lining here: save time on getting ready. Makeup on, plop on wig, and I'm ready to go.

Looking at all the wigs, I realize this will be my new normal. I WILL HAVE NO HAIR. This wig will be my new look. Will I like wearing it? Many warriors who have gone before me have told me they hated wearing a wig. They resorted to scarves or even going bald. It empowered them. Will I feel the same?

I begin trying on the wigs. I try a long blonde wig—NO! Next is a black Cleopatra-type wig—NO! I try on one with long hair that flips—it's okay but not me. Debbie has been helping immensely. Bob is giving his opinion and picking out wigs for me to try. We're having *fun*.

We all agree on two. Both have my coloring; one in the style I wear now and one a little shorter. And they look like real hair—score! When Debbie comes to my house to shave my head, she'll style my wigs.

Could I have anyone kinder in my life? A generous loving soul. *See the gifts cancer is giving me?*

Pamela explains the care of my wigs. While wearing it, I'm never to open a hot oven or dryer as the steam could melt it. No longer having to get clothes out of the dryer? Bonus! I'm to bring my wig to her once a month for cleaning. Information given, ready to go.

I have a script for a *cranial prosthetic* and am told to never ever say wig when submitting my claim or the insurance will not cover the cost. Really? They'll pay for chemo but not the wig you need because of the side effects? I will never understand insurance companies.

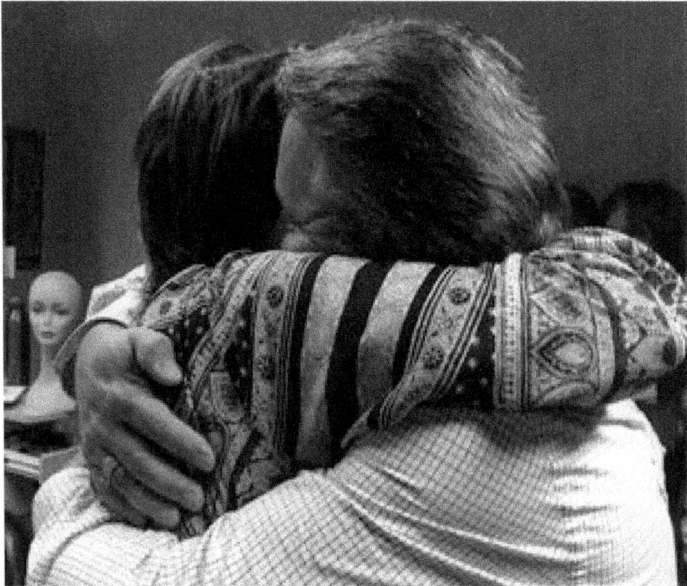

We spend $1,000 on two wigs. I look at my husband when I see the bill. His response? "The cost means nothing; I will pay any price, so you feel good about yourself." We end with a hug. A hug filled with love, support, relief, and for accomplishing another step in the journey together. It was perfect.

> *I have learned there is more power in a good strong hug*
> *than in a thousand meaningful words.*
> —Ann Hood

The Marriage of the Two
June 27th

My plan is to use both traditional and integrative medicine while treating the Big "C". I have an appointment today with Dr. Michael Walker, a naturopath oncologist from the Integrative Medicine Department. (Maureen's recommendation.) As a naturopath, he will give me recommendations of natural treatments which will help me through chemo and its side effects. Nothing he advises will interfere with anything I am going to have through traditional medicine. A win-win in my book.

When Maureen told me about him, she said he looks young, but don't let that fool you, he's excellent in his job (and I find out she's right). Young? He walks in and all I can think of is "Doogie Howser." Honestly, he looks like he's fresh out of high school. *(I'm dying to ask his age.)* Putting my trust in Maureen, we begin with my cancer history. I give him the rundown on both 'dances,' ending with my current treatment plan and my worry about chemo side effects. I ask him how he feels, as a naturopath oncologist, about the chemicals used in chemotherapy. After a lengthy discussion, we agree it's the proven treatment for cancer.

Yes, the cancer was removed with the mastectomy but to guarantee no rogue cells have gone elsewhere, the chemo will cover my entire body to kill off any 'runners.' He says it's like a dandelion. If it's yellow and you remove the plant, root, and all, from the ground it won't come back. But if the dandelion is white with all the seeds, when you remove the weed, the white fluffy seeds fly everywhere. The chemo is just guaranteeing I've taken care of any white fluffies. (Okay, he didn't say white fluffies, but it works for me.)

Diet has a significant impact on quality of life, especially during chemo. The oncology nurse told me there is no diet to follow; they just want me to eat. I laugh and tell him there may be a bonus here, losing weight. He tells me the opposite; studies show body mass helps with chemo. He doesn't want me to lose a lot of weight. I'll admit I have no trouble in the body mass department, so I'm set there.

He wants me to follow the Mediterranean diet and gives me a list of foods. Part of the diet is eating oily fish 3 times a week. This might be a problem as I don't like sardines or anchovies. *Yuck!* I keep looking over the list. I'm in luck there's salmon. I agree to eat it as least twice a week. The rest of the time I'll eat chicken with red meat occasionally. He gives me information about a study in Spain which found following a Mediterranean diet can prevent reoccurrence. *Well, then, I'm in.*

He explains the side effects of chemo: nausea and fatigue being the main ones. (*Yep, like a broken record.*) I can never get away from those two. It seems they'll be with me throughout the journey. Chemo could have an effect on my heart. (*Seriously, they can't invent a chemo that doesn't damage the heart?*) He puts me on three different supplements: Ultra Omega-3, a probiotic, and UBQH to help my heart. I'm to begin taking them before I start chemo. I guess I'm a pill popper now, something new for me.

I want to know what treatments will help me with chemo side effects. Like Maureen, he suggests acupuncture the day before the chemo. It will help with the nausea. I'm not sure when I should have a Reiki treatment: before, during or after treatment. The answer: Any time I receive it will be beneficial. Further on down the line, oncology massage and guided imagery will also help.

He reiterates what Dr. Hanna and his oncology nurse have told me. Exercise is helpful while going through treatment. Even if it's a small walk a day, it's beneficial. Swimming will be an excellent way to keep up my energy levels. When I get home, I'm ordering a mastectomy suit from Land's End so when I get the green light to swim, I'm ready. Who knew they made such a thing? Thank you, Land's End.

Dr. Walker tells me he will be working with Dr. Hanna on my treatment plan and seeing me through the end of radiation. That comforts me; I have another expert on my side, someone else who has knowledge to help me navigate through this. I'm feeling optimistic!

> *Positivity always wins, always.*
> —Gary Vaynerchuk

Getting my Ducks in a Row
June 27th – July 6th

My chemo is to begin on July 12th. I begin to get things done for the next phase of my journey.

I finish plans for the wedding, which is August 18th. I'm glad to do this. Nick's wedding has helped me focus on something other than cancer. I purchase my dress (navy) I didn't do the requisite mother of the groom beige. Finalize the menus for the rehearsal dinner and after brunch. The list of songs for the band is done. I've written out what I want done for all wedding events in case I get chemo brain and forget something. Wedding plans done. Check!

I have met with Dr. Walker and am instituting his suggestions, taking the vitamins and other supplements he ordered. Blood work has been done so we can track my progress. I set an appointment for acupuncture to offset any chemo side effects. I know he is a phone call away if I need help.

Wigs bought and scarves ordered. Purchased ginger ale, ginger hard candies, food I think I'll like to eat. I recorded a gazillion movies and TV shows to watch and downloaded books on my Kindle.

I've reinstated my gym membership to swim during chemo. Keeping my fingers crossed it helps with my energy levels. Besides, I miss my lady friends immensely.

I'm diligently using the EES on my eyebrows twice a day to hopefully prevent their loss. Arnica cream is put on my scars. I'm walking daily to keep up my energy.

I get my teeth cleaned because I know I won't be able to for a while. The dental hygienist is going through Stage 2 breast cancer. She shares her stories. For the first time, hearing someone else's story doesn't bother me. Instead, I find it comforting.

105

I've met with Natalie to help me process what's about to happen. I meditate and manifest daily. My mindset is this is going to be trying at times but doable. Just another part of the job of healing.

I'm doing all this to hopefully make this journey surmountable. I'm in the unknown. I have no idea how I will handle this until I go through it and not knowing is killing me. I have to remember patience; that everyone has their own unique journey and to stay in the NOW. And the most important thing to remember? No matter how my body handles this, chemo is allowing me to have a longer life. Gratitude. Yep, there's a silver lining here and I just found it.

> *In every dark cloud there is a silver lining. To find the silver lining in your challenges, shift your perspective.*
> —Unknown

The Chemo Moon
July 7th – 9th

Before I begin chemo, I want to go away with my husband. You know how couples go on a 'babymoon' before they have a baby, I wanted a 'chemo moon.' I had no idea what I was getting into. When would be the next time I would feel great? We plan a trip to northern Michigan.

I have an 8:30 appointment to check my mastectomy scar to ensure its healing. Theresa examines me first. She's concerned about two pinpoints. She tells me they may not let me begin my chemo if they aren't closed. The area where she has concerns is where my bra has been rubbing. *Say what?*

Dr. Ruark comes in next. She's also concerned. *Really Universe. I do not want to delay this.* She wants me to inform my oncologist and come back on Tuesday to take another look before she gives me the go-ahead to begin chemo. She suggests wearing gauze to cover the area or not wear a bra. Not wear a bra? *Yikes!* I leave concerned I'm not going to be able to start my chemo on time. I don't want anything to jeopardize my schedule.

I leave a message with my oncologist, letting them know what my surgeon has said. I don't hear back. I take that as good news.

Our friends John and Cindy (Go Gypsy Vodka) have graciously offered to let us stay with them on Crooked Lake and we readily accept the offer. I want to be in Harbor Springs/Petoskey. I think it's one of the most beautiful places in Michigan, it's my happy place.

The sun is out, and the sky is blue when we arrive, Pure Michigan. John and Cindy take us on a boat ride, and all is right with the world. The next morning, we head into Harbor Springs, walk around town, and visit my favorite spots. Rejuvenized, we head to Mackinac Island.

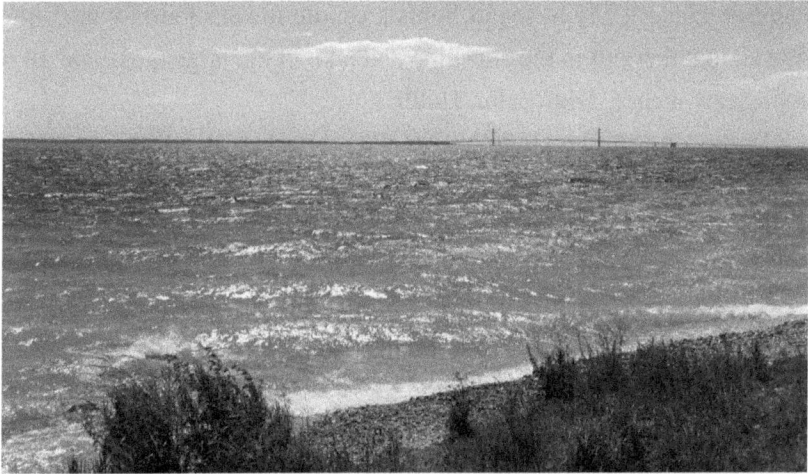

The weather is perfect, the scenery stunning. Getting away was the best idea. The Island House is a beautiful hotel with a fantastic view. We walk, explore, and take in the energy of the water and find peace. Bottom line: We had fun and forgot about life for a while. *Perfection.*

Neither of us are in a rush to get home. We seem to want to delay it because we know once there, reality hits. While driving, I mentioned I want to stop in Indian River to visit the Cross in the Woods Shrine. (www.crossinthewoods.com) I **need** to go. I've never been there before, but I want to pray and meditate.

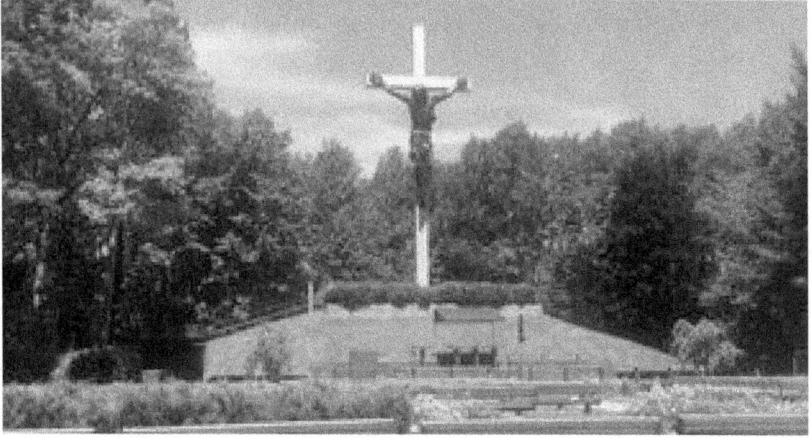

It's everything I hoped it would be. Pure peace. We walk the meditation trail and pray in the small chapel to St. Peregrine (patron saint of cancer). My husband lights a candle for our journey to come. We sit together out in the sunshine and take in the large cross and all it represents. Peace, faith, calm, HOPE.

We're home around 6:00 p.m. feeling refreshed and ready to take on the next phase.

> *Hope is the companion of power, and mother of success;*
> *for who so hopes strongly has within him the gift of miracles.*
> —Samuel Smiles

Pin Cushion Time!
July 10th

I've taken Dr. Walker's recommendation and make an appointment for an acupuncture treatment. This will help with chemo side effects, most specifically, nausea. Feeling nauseous 24/7 doesn't appeal to me, so any help I can get, sign me up.

It's a rainy day. A day where you want to stay in bed. I'm a little apprehensive about needles being stuck in me, but if it will help with the side effects, I'll suck it up.

The integrative medicine area is like a spa. Quiet music, aromatherapy, a pure Zen vibe. The room I'm in has muted lighting with a heated massage table. It does help calm me. I meet the acupuncturist, and we begin. She explains the concept of acupuncture. Acupuncture is the insertion of very fine needles in various points on the body's surface to influence physiological functioning of the body. Acupuncture mobilizes and regulates qi and blood to invigorate the physiological function of the muscles, nerves, glands and organs.

Fun fact: When I ask her how long the needles will stay inserted. She explains the length of time depends on the time of year. Since it's summer and we just had the summer solstice, the needles will not need to stay in as long. It has to do with the Earth's pressure. I'm silently thankful it's summer.

The needles are small. (That helps my nerves.) She begins by placing two on each calf. I feel a tiny poke, really nothing at all. She proceeds to put one on the top of each foot. One goes in the top of my head and finally one in each ear. She tells me the ones placed in the ears will help with anxiety and stress. (*Um—can she just keep those in my ears permanently?*) I don't feel them once they're in.

She turns on meditative music and leaves. Laying there, I think about my journey ahead, how I'm taking time for self-care to prepare me for the next phase of my healing. It's been foreign to me to put myself first. I think this is one of the most valuable lessons I'm learning on this journey, *to love me*. I eventually fall into a deep sleep and wake up when the acupuncturist comes in. I feel calm and rested.

She tells me it may take a few sessions; very few people get 100% improvement on the first visit. It's a buildup effect. I've decided to schedule appointments before each chemo treatment. Every little bit helps is my motto. Onward and upward!

Fall in love with caring for yourself, in body, mind and spirit.
—Jenni Cornette

A Much-Needed Tune-Up
(or Talk Carey Off the Wall)
July 11th

Cancer challenges you both physically and mentally. Each time I've been diagnosed with the Big "C" the medical community has been quick to set up appointments with health care professionals to help me heal my physical self, but it has not addressed my emotional well-being. Having been through this dance twice, I know there is a need to help patients heal mentally.

Each life experience, even those which are not positive, are still gifts. I come away with deeper insight and growth. By staying grateful, when the difficult experiences present themselves, they became less dramatic and much easier to get through. It's during those times when I've worked hard to find the gratitude, I find serenity. Navigating my way through cancer with gratitude has helped make it a journey of peace. But that does not mean I don't get overwhelmed.

When I was diagnosed the second time, I once again turned to Natalie. I knew this journey was going to be more intense; my diagnosis was more serious. I was on overload.

I purposely set an appointment with her for the day before my first chemo treatment. I'm mentally a mess, the fear of the unknown is taking over. I have no idea what's ahead. *Was I going to be deathly ill, throwing up all the time? Will I to be so exhausted I can't function? Will the procedure itself hurt?* AHHHH! I need a "tune-up."

Natalie asks what I'm feeling. Scared, sad, apprehensive, overwhelmed about the next steps of my journey. One thing which comes out in our discussion is my need for control. I want to be in control of something which is uncontrollable.

I've done all I can do to get ready for this. As my friend Becky pointed out, I've used my fear to prepare myself. I've met with several doctors and medical personnel to discuss my treatment plan. Completed all medical procedures required. I prepared myself for the physical changes I'll experience. Yet, I still have **no** power over what's going to happen to me, yet I *want* to control this.

I tell Natalie about my phone calls with Riley. She's sad she's not here with me and worried about chemo. I remind her there will be times I'll be tired and not feeling well. How she needs to remember this is just the chemo working and doing its job. That this is temporary.

Natalie asks me if I can remember this for myself when I'm going through it. Can I realize it's temporary? Can I just go with the flow? Embrace the chemo for what it's giving me? I think about this and respond, "Bottom line, I don't want to do this." Yes, I know that's not a possibility, but there are times when I feel like I'm in a nightmare and miraculously I'll wake up and it's all been a bad dream.

We continue to talk, and I realize I've let fear consume me. After more discussion, I say, yes, I'll go with the flow. It will be extremely difficult for me. I will have to work hard at this. But she's right. Trying to control this and anticipate the unknown is driving me crazy. *Let it go. Let it flow, Carey.*

It's like I'm in a constant mental battle during this journey, trying to keep myself out of the dark. After much thought, I again realize how important it is to stay present. I'm conjuring up scenarios which don't serve me. And the most important thing I really need to remember is no matter what my side effects are *it is what it is*, and I will just handle it. It's *temporary*. Thank you, Natalie.

> *If you can't control the current of the river, then just go with the flow.*
> —Unknown

Relishing the Moment
July 11ᵗʰ—Later That Day

After my session with Natalie, I have an appointment with the breast surgeon. (On a side note: to not jeopardize my chemo start date, I didn't wear a bra all weekend. I wear a bulky jacket, and no one can tell. *Whoop! Whoop! Winning.)*

As Theresa is examining me to see if my chest has thoroughly healed, she tells me the pinpoints have cleared but now she sees a rash on my stomach. She thinks it may be a yeast infection. If it is, it could delay my chemo. *Seriously?*

This is **not** what I want to hear. The pinpoints are closed and now this? I don't want to jeopardize my chemo schedule as my focus is on my son's wedding. We agree I will apply cortisone to the area and call my oncology nurse. I leave hopeful but apprehensive.

Later, we go to Denise's for a family dinner. It's nice to have a diversion. We forget about tomorrow for a while. We're in bed by 11:30, Bob is asleep immediately, of course. I, on the other hand, watch television and eventually read.

It's close to 3:30 and I'm still not sleeping. Bob wakes up and asks if I'm all right. "Yes, I respond, just fine." "Then why aren't you asleep?" He asks. I start to cry and say, "I don't want to go to sleep. I want to stay awake and feel normal for a while longer. I'm not in pain. I don't feel fatigued or nauseous. I have my hair. I don't know when I'll feel like this again. I don't want to let it go. I want to relish this moment." He understands and holds me until I eventually fall asleep.

> *Take life day by day and be grateful for the little things.*
> *Don't get stressed over what you can't control.*
> —Unknown

Chemotherapy—The Red Devil

And So, It Begins

July 12th

I wake up, ground myself, and meditate. I find my gratitude for what I'm to be given today. I'm going with the flow and accepting what the world will bring. I apply a glob of the lidocaine cream on my port and cover it with Saran Wrap an hour before arrival, keeping my fingers crossed it works. We pack our bags and we're ready to go.

On the way, I listen to my go-to station on Pandora. All my favorite songs are playing on the way—even my all-time favorite—'September.' I dance in the car. Isn't it the best happy song?

Arriving 10 minutes early, we walk in silence and get in the elevator. A woman comes in with her husband. A cancer patient, she has a scarf covering her bald head and is grinning from ear to ear. She's exuding happiness. She's going to Floor 3. She looks at me and says, "Going to Floor 2?" I nod yes. She smiles and says, "I'll be there soon too. Have a wonderful day." Wow, what a gift she was to me! A smiling angel on Earth. Seeing her happy helped me feel peace.

I arrive on Floor 2 and walk into the infusion center. This is so surreal for me. I've walked into this place for the past three years to administer Reiki and now **I'm** the patient. I check in, sign all the consent forms, and get my wristband. Hanna, an aide, brings me back to the infusion area. When I walk in, I say hello to some of the nurses. They're surprised to see me and greet me with hugs. I'm fighting back tears. I'm not feeling too brave right now.

I'm going to be in the last bay. Hannah gives me a choice of cubicles. I choose the one with more privacy versus windows. Anna is to be my nurse today. She knows me and immediately puts me at ease. I'm worried about the IV being inserted into the port. She says I've put the lidocaine cream on correctly so I shouldn't feel anything. Whew! I'm relaxing a little bit more. Notice I said a *bit*.

Before we begin, Anna explains the different drugs I will receive during each infusion and how long the infusion will last. I've heard this before, but in this moment, I remember nothing, so I'm glad to hear it again. I will have two anti-nausea meds, Pepcid, Benadryl, and a steroid before she administers the actual chemo. I will receive two different chemo drugs followed by a saline flush.

Time to see if the lidocaine really works. I turn my head to the left when Anna begins. *So not watching this!* I feel nothing when she inserts the needle. It did take two tries but it's in and I'm wired to go.

She begins with an anti-nausea medication. She injects it directly into the IV. A second bag is dripped in, it's Pepcid for my stomach, followed by another bag of anti-nausea meds. Next is the Benadryl. My head gets cloudy, and I feel tired when it is given to me. And finally, the steroid. Once those are finished, Anna places the order to the pharmacy for my chemo drugs. The premeds have taken an hour. I rest and wait for them to be delivered.

While waiting, two nurses come over to see me. Bernie is a nurse to whom I've administered Reiki. She immediately hugs me and tells me I'm going to be just fine. She brings tears to my eyes. I'm having a difficult time not crying today. I'm feeling the love from these incredible women, and it humbles me. I'm happy with my decision to have my chemo administered here. I feel at home.

My chemo has arrived. The first drug, Adriamycin, is injected by Anna. It's in two huge syringes and I mean HUGE. The bag that brings the vials has a large hazardous sign on it. *I really didn't need to see that.* I find out later from Renee that my husband is texting her throughout the process, and he's freaking out when he sees it.

Anna must administer it slowly as I could get very nauseous. This chemo is nicknamed the "Red Devil" and after seeing the hazardous sign on the packaging, I can believe it. The process takes 30 minutes. I'm warned again my urine will be red the first few times I go to the bathroom and to not let it alarm me. Red Devil complete, it's time for the final chemo drug, cyclophosphamide. This will be administered via a drip bag and will take an hour.

One of the bonuses during an infusion is the warm blankets. Hanna is great. She checks on me often and always makes sure I have ice water, graham crackers, and many warm blankets.

Under the warmth of the blankets, I fall asleep for the last hour. I sleep peacefully probably from the lack of sleep from the night before. I wake up and Anna gives me one more flush of saline. It makes me feel a little nauseous. I pop in an Altoid; the peppermint helps.

I'm to have an injection of Neulasta within 24 hours of treatment. The chemo I'm receiving depletes my immune system so the Neulasta will help protect me from an infection. I can either come in tomorrow and receive the injection or they can put a patch on my arm, which has a timer and will inject me at the appropriate time.

The wimp in me originally says no to the patch. I didn't want to have to worry about something stuck on my arm. My husband, once again, helps me see the logic. Sitting at home relaxing or driving back to the hospital, fighting traffic, parking, waiting, etc., logic wins out. Anna puts on the patch. It has a sticky backing and starts to tick as when she puts it on. It ticks for about 15 seconds then I feel a pop. I'm assuming that was the needle going in, but then I prefer to not think about that. Patch in place, good to go. Bob and I walk to the elevator, do a happy dance and hug. This is doable, this is tolerable. I'm grateful for today. One treatment down—15 to go. *Whoop! Whoop!*

> *Accomplishments give you a sense of confidence and encouragement.*
> —Catherine Pulsifer

Roller-Coaster Ride
July 12th—Later that Day

I'm home from my treatment spending the day relaxing and watching one of the gazillion movies I've recorded. I faithfully take my anti-nausea medication even though I'm not feeling too nauseous. I have a good appetite when I get home and eat chicken noodle soup along with a PB&J. I'm thinking, *"This is fine. I can do this."* Then dinnertime rolls around. Yep, the chicken soup that tasted so good at lunch; I can't stand the smell of it. Is this what dogs go through? I think I've become part dog! My smelling capabilities have just intensified 1,000%.

The only thing that sounds remotely appetizing is a bagel. Bob gets me one and I can eat half. So, this is what they mean when they say the chemo diet. If this continues, I may have to order a smaller size dress for the wedding—*BONUS. Yep, I'm always looking for the silver lining.*

> *To many people miss the silver lining because they're expecting gold.*
> —Maurice Setter

Getting Into the Swing of Things
July 14th – 15th

Although the first night took a lot out of me, for the next few days, I make sure I walk to keep up my stamina.

I wake up the next two mornings around 4:30 extremely nauseous. It feels like morning sickness combined with a hangover. *Yuck! And I didn't even get to have fun to feel this way.* I immediately take anti-nausea meds and drink a ton of water. Of course, I can't fall back asleep. My sleep patterns are off, but overall, this is doable.

> *I have the attitude that anything is doable, I can make anything happen.*
> —Lori Greiner

The Tsunami Hits
July 16th

It's Saturday morning and I wake up violently ill. I've never felt so nauseous. It scares me. My ever-present knight in shining armor, Bob, asks what he can do to help me. Would I like something to eat? I'm fighting off tears (really if I start, I'm not sure I'll be able to stop) and say yes, a bagel. He's gotten me cinnamon raisin muffins, which I usually love, but just thinking of eating a raisin makes me queasy.

It's 6:30 in the morning and he rushes to Tim Horton's to get me a toasted bagel. Seriously, is he not the best man around? I eat the bagel, drink some Vernors Ginger Ale (it's a Michigan thing). We lie back in bed, hold hands, and fall asleep for three hours. Pure bliss. I love sleeping; I don't feel sick, and it allows me to escape for a while.

I find today I'm more exhausted than I was yesterday. I'm into Day 4. I walk the perimeter of my home to get in some exercise, but I find this tires me. (I live on an acre of land so it's not a short walk.) I have to take Bob to pick up Riley's car and am exhausted when I get home. I figure the days immediately following an infusion will be the days I need to conserve my energy. This is trial-and-error time. Flowing with the unknown. Observing how my body will manage this. Keeping myself a little cocooned to stay healthy.

Denise has stopped by and brings me chicken soup. During our visit, I tell her how many people have touched my life during this. It's amazing to me really. Our cousin Anne-Marie sends me a card every week. Receiving them brightens my day and it touches my heart that she's taking time to do this for me.

A cousin of Bob's, Meri Cornacchini, who lives in Italy, whom I've never met, gives me uplifting messages on Facebook. Friends from over 40 years ago are reaching out to give me encouragement. I've received endless messages, cards, flowers, and meals, I'm surrounded with love.

I may be feeling physically low today, but how can I let it get me down when I'm cocooned by this loving energy? I feel it and it gives me hope. This is difficult, but I refuse to look at that way; when I'm journeying through this in love and gratitude.

> *Gratitude is the shortcut which speeds the journey to love.*
> —Raymond D. Longoria

Little Things
July 18th

Last night Bob and I were watching television when he looked over and I had tears in my eyes. Looking concerned, he asked if I was in pain. I said, "No, I was just running my fingers through my hair and relishing the fact I can still do this." It's funny something so normal we take for granted could mean so much to me. Trust me, it's not like I have great hair. Think fine and thin when describing it, but nonetheless, it's my mine and I'm going to lose it.

I've been told my head will begin to feel tingly before my hair begins to fall out. It's supposed to happen 14 days after my first treatment, which means it will be before my next treatment on Wednesday, July 26th. I ponder what I'll look like.

It's an odd feeling to know you're going to lose your hair. Rationally, I know this is going to happen, but mentally am I prepared for this? I think losing my hair will really drive home that I have cancer. Silly, isn't it? I've had my breast removed and started chemo, yet I don't feel like I have cancer. I know it's not rational. I think about this and realize that if you look at me, I don't look sick.

What is cancer supposed to look like? I don't look gaunt; my skin coloring is good, and I have my hair. I can camouflage my missing breast, I can wear makeup to cover any paleness, but my hair? Every time I look in the mirror, I will see this. I will see a new me—a bald version. Will I feel empowered, angry, sad?

I find myself touching my hair and enjoying the moments I have left of little things—washing, drying, combing, curling. I put it in a ponytail and am happy I'm able to do this. *Little things.*

I wonder how much more of my physical body I will have to sacrifice. Isn't it bad enough I have cancer? I already gave up my breast. Do I have to give up my hair, too? And when thinking about it, the answer is **yes**. Yes, I do and it's a small price to pay to *live*. I need to change my mindset and focus on the big picture. I've readily given up my breast to rid myself of cancer. I've chosen to have the chemo to help me live a longer life. Sacrificing my hair is a part of that decision.

Cancer can have my hair, but it can't have ME. I watched a video of a woman shaving her head during her second bout with cancer. She said something so profound which helped me immensely. "Shaving my head, losing my hair is what HEALING looks like." I am healing, that's all, and this is a part of the process.

I'll shave my head when the time comes and embrace the moment. But for now, I'll relish the little things like playing with my hair.

> *Sometimes, Pooh said, the smallest things take up the most room in your heart.*
> —Winnie the Pooh

Buying Texas
July 21st

Before my diagnosis, I had been going to Lifetime Fitness five days a week to do water aerobics. I was in the best physical shape I'd been in a while, so I had great energy going into this journey. I haven't been able to get in the pool since May 31st; I'm dying to get back. Walking every day isn't the same. I miss swimming and my lady friends. It has been frustrating waiting—waiting to heal, waiting for the first chemo. **Waiting!** (*What is it with cancer and waiting?*)

Anticipating I would eventually get the go-ahead, I bought a mastectomy suit from Lands' End. Suit bought, but what do I put in it? I can't wear a suit with just *one* breast. That would just look weird. Flat on one side, a breast on the other. Nope, that won't do. Do they even make prosthetics for the water? I called Image Recovery and found out there is such a thing. *Whoo-hoo!* Appointment made, bathing suit in hand, I head over.

In the fitting room checking out the silicone prosthetics, they look like giant jellyfish, clear blobs. Does my real breast look like this? I get over the 'look' of the prosthetic and move on to the size—*gargantuan*. I swear when I get the new set, they're going to be B's. I reach out and grab one. It's huge, squishy, and HEAVY. Truly, can't I just catch a break? I'll be swimming with a weight on. Will I swim lopsided? I've got to put this thing on a scale when I get home.

Mastectomy suits have a slit on the side where you can slip in the prosthetic. (Obviously, the makers of the suit must assume everyone is an A cup by the size of the slit.) I begin to attempt to put the 'jellyfish' into my suit. The meaning of attempt: *make an effort to achieve or complete something, typically a difficult task or action.* That would about sum up what I was doing, attempting a difficult task. It was like trying to stuff an elephant into a mouse hole.

Short of calling in the Calvary, after much pushing and shoving, I finally get it in. I look in the mirror, looking straight on, turning from side to side. I have no idea if this is the correct one. I finally ask for help. This is where the "breast cancer has no dignity" thing comes in. I have exposed myself to more strangers than I care to remember.

Once again, a stranger is feeling me up and looking at my chest. She assesses me and says, "I think it's too small, you need a bigger size." Are you kidding me? The next size must be as big as the state of Texas!

She grabs a larger size, and we attempt (*remember the meaning*) to take out the smaller size and replace it with the larger one. It wasn't just me. She finds it difficult also. After much struggling, she finally gets Texas in, and I turn to look in the mirror. OMG—It does look better. I purchase Texas along with a few hats for good measure and head home. I'm feeling optimistic about swimming.

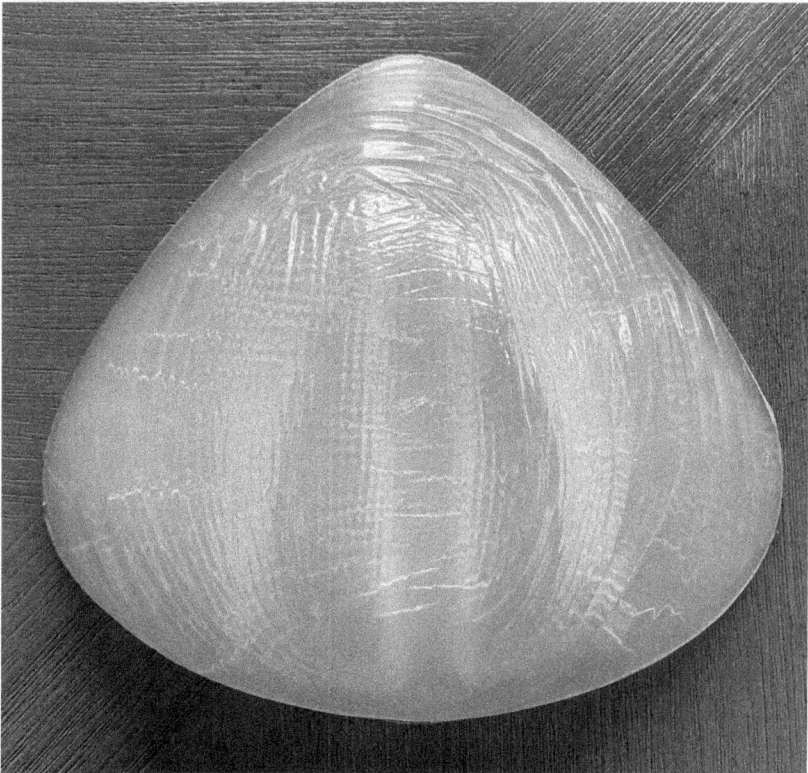

I see my oncologist, Dr. Hanna, that afternoon. He normally sees me after each chemo treatment. He says I'm handling it so well I won't need to see him for a month. I ask if I can begin swimming. The answer? *YES*. Being told I'm handling chemo well and getting permission to start swimming was Double *Whoop! Whoop!* Today is a great day, Texas and all.

> *Every day is a good day, there is something to learn, care and celebrate.*
> —Amit Ray

Trying Out Texas
July 22nd

I wake up looking forward to the day. I get to swim! I'm still nauseous, but it's tolerable. I eat breakfast, grab Texas, and miraculously insert it in my suit. I'm ready to go.

The closer I get to Lifetime, the happier I am. I arrive and walk in with my friend Tina. This feels normal. I walk into class and am greeted by John, the instructor. I show him Texas and ask, "What do you think? I wonder if I'll float, or do you think it will weigh me down?" He laughs. John gets me.

I get into the water and feel at home. I'm doing something normal today and I feel great. I work out the entire hour, though there are times when I need to pace myself. John gives me instructions, so I won't damage anything, but I did it! I feel energized. Despite chemo, I did something normal. On the way home, I get a smoothie and think to myself, "Today is another great day, Texas and all!"

> *I think it's important to find the little things in everyday life that make you happy.*
> —Paula Cole

Hair Today, Gone Tomorrow—A New Normal
July 27th

Not having hair makes me feel like it's a neon sign flashing, *"Look she has cancer."* Everyone will know. Even though friends and family know I have cancer, I prefer the world not see me any differently. I don't want special treatment or looks of shock or pity. I don't have the energy to answer questions. I just want to go about my life while treating the Big "C".

One of Riley's concerns when she left for Barcelona was how I would look when she comes home. Losing my hair upsets her immensely. She will be home this Sunday. To prepare her I mentioned during one of our FaceTime chats that my hair will be gone soon. She starts crying and so do I. (I hate seeing my kids upset—*Thanks cancer.*) We talk and I remind her this is a part of the healing process. Chemo is doing its job and, the most important thing, this is temporary. (*I seem to always be reminding myself of this.*)

I tell her again how I don't want to pull my hair out in clumps. I'd rather be in control. She understands but is so frustrated this is happening. To lighten the mood, I tell her dad is excited, he thinks I'll look exotic. She laughs. I say, "I know. Weird, right?" Riley set, now on to taking care of me.

Like clockwork, 14 days after my first chemo it starts. On Tuesday, I go swimming and, in the shower, as I'm washing my hair, strands come out. Later at home, when I run my fingers through my hair, more strands. It has begun. The next part of the process is here. My hair will be gone in the next few days. I will have a new normal. No hair until next year. I will have what my dad used to call a 'baldy sour'—*OMG.*

Time to look at the bright side, Carey. Getting ready just got slashed in half. I will no longer have to do my hair (something I hate doing and suck at). Bad hair days are gone. I won't have to shave my legs—*score.* No more chin hairs, really? (And who invented those anyway?) I hear your hair comes back thick and curly, *double score.* And once again, this is all **temporary**.

I'll shave my hair in the next few days and create a new normal. Life as a cancer patient, always creating a new normal.

> ***Brave is finding a new normal.***
> —Gina Lapapa

This Is What Healing Looks Like
July 30th

I decided to shave my head today. Debbie, my beautician, graciously offered to come to my home and shave it for me. *What a gift.* I originally scheduled it for Thursday, but Bob looked at me and said, "Your hair looks fine, why not wait until the weekend?" I, of course, wanted to have my hair as long as I could, so today will be the day.

The timeframe for losing my hair was spot on. Like clockwork on Day 14, I would thread my fingers through my hair and large strands would come out. Today it was coming out in clumps. I was ready.

In all honesty, I was feeling sad. Shaving my head was another cancer wake-up call, another reality check.

How would it physically feel? Would my head be extra sensitive? What will my head be shaped like? Would I always be cold? So many questions running through my mind.

I take my hair products: hair dryer, curling iron, and hairbrushes and reverently put them away. I won't be needing them for a while. I'm sad while doing this; realizing what will happen today.

Washing my hair for the last time, I embraced the moment, knowing it will be a long time before I do this again. *Moments.* That's what cancer gives you. Moments to store away and savor.

Riley came home this morning from Barcelona, so no matter what was happening to me today, it was a great day.

Debbie came over at 3 p.m. We visited for a while, which was what I needed. After some discussion, we decide to trim my hair first then shave it, instead of outright shaving it. I'm so glad we made that decision. I got to relish feeling Debbie's fingers through my hair while getting my last haircut. Haircut done—on to shaving my head.

Debbie begins by giving me a kiss, my husband holding my hand with Riley standing next to me. I was going through something heartbreaking, but I was feeling nothing but love. She gently shaves it away. My hair is gone, but I have a precious memory.

I am supported during this journey. I am loved. I am once again in gratitude. Cancer can try to take things away from me, but it can't take away love, it can't take away memories, it can't take away **me**. Because deep down, even though my body has been through hell, I no longer have a breast or hair, I'm still me. A little altered but still me.

I debated on whether I should share the picture of my new do as it's as raw as it gets; but when I began this dance with the Big "C", I told myself to keep it real. No holds barred. I wanted to let you in on my journey—warts and all. The picture I'm sharing is not one of a cancer patient who has just lost her hair, but a picture that shows what unconditional love and healing looks like and I think it's beautiful.

> *I show my scars so others can know they can heal.*
> —Racheffe Nicole

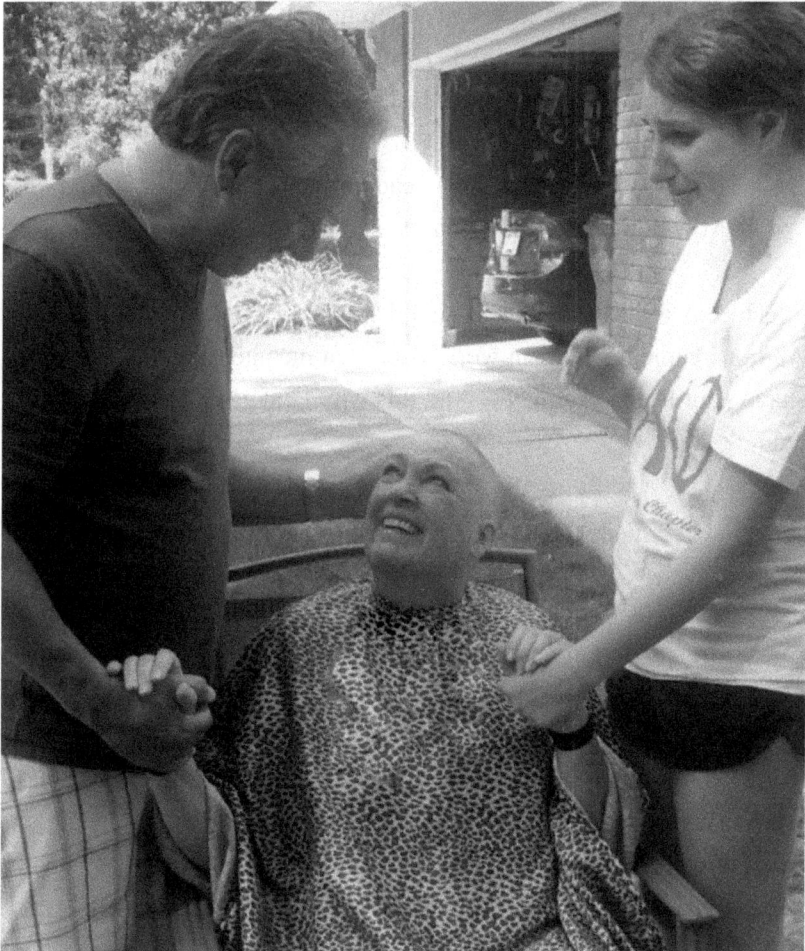

Quick Thoughts on Having No Hair

- I feel cooler. Hot flashes have now been taken down a notch or two. *Bonus!*
- I wear a little beanie to bed as my head does get cold.
- I have a good-shaped head. It's not as small as I thought.
- My head was sensitive the first few days until all my hair was gone.
- I look horrendous in hats. I've decided that hats look best when you can have little hair wisps coming out the side.
- I sometimes forget that I've shaved my head until I walk by a mirror, and look and say to myself, "Who are you?"
- Showers are much quicker since there's no hair to wash.
- The time to get ready has just been slashed in half.
- I never have a bad hair day.
- Bob constantly kisses my head and tells me I'm beautiful.
- My children have all seen me and are fine with it.

The day after I shaved my head, I was wearing my new wig. Anthony came home from work, looked at me and said, "Didn't you shave your head yesterday?" And this why God gave me Anthony, comic relief.

> *I show my scars so others can know they can heal.*
> —Racheffe Nicole

And So, It Goes
August 9th

Today is my third chemo treatment. I never sleep the night before as I want to relish my body feeling well. I know once I have my chemo, the cycle will begin again. Fatigue and nausea. It's the nausea that gets me. I know this is a by-product of the chemo and I'm bracing for it.

I sometimes have a pity party for myself when I'm going through chemo. I had a meltdown last time when I was in the thick of it, crying to Bob I was tired of it all. I've lost a breast, lost my hair and am so tired of being nauseous. I tell him I can't wait for the day when I wake up feeling good. It's exhausting treating cancer and some days I'm just that—exhausted. I get apprehensive about going to chemo. Not for the actual process, it's a breeze, but for the side effects I will feel for the next two weeks.

I'm especially nervous for this chemo as I have had a cold. I freaked out on Sunday because I was worried about my system being compromised already going into this chemo. Nicholas is getting married on August 18th. I have 10 days from this chemo to feel better. What if my cold gets worse? I call my oncology nurse on Monday and ask her to 'talk-me off the ledge.' My only concern is the wedding. She orders a Z-Pak for me, and it puts me at ease. *Whoop! Whoop!*

It's 8:00 in the morning. I'm writing to ease my mind. I know this is all doable. I know I will be uncomfortable for a few days, but I will get through it. I have an end goal in mind—the wedding. I am reminding myself I signed up for this, side effects and all. I need to focus on the goal. Yes, the timing sucks. I would have rather not been going through treatments during this special time for us. I would like my body to be at 100%. But in the grand scheme of things, I get to be at my son's wedding. How lucky and blessed am I?

I will gladly receive my chemo. It's a gift I shouldn't wish away. It is giving me life and I'm thankful for it.

> *Sometimes you just have to put your big girl panties and deal with it.*
> —Unknown

The Wedding Song
August 18th

Looking back, the timing of Nick's wedding was a godsend. It gave me something to focus on besides cancer. The wedding was everything I'd hoped it would be for Nick and Molly. Molly was a beautiful bride. The weather was perfect, the food was excellent, the band was great, everyone danced, the atmosphere was loving and celebratory. It was a true celebration of love.

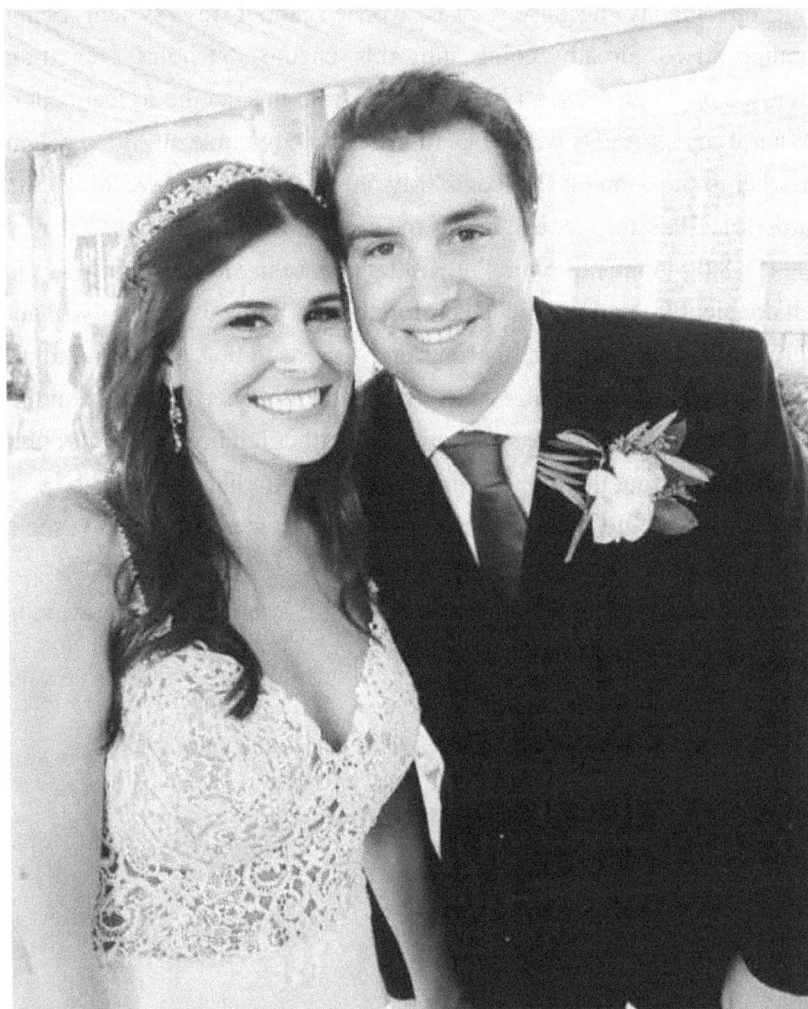

When Nick announced he was getting married, all my girlfriends, who had sons, told me two things. As the mother of the groom, you're supposed to wear beige and stay quiet, and there would be one point during the wedding which would be your special moment—the mother/son dance. Make it magical, they said. Make sure you pick a song that will resonate with your son.

The pressure was on. I immediately went on the internet and began searching. During this frantic search for the most perfect song, I had an aha moment: Nick's a guy, he could care less what song I pick. If you ask him the day after the wedding what we danced to, his response is going to be, "I don't know, some song." Once I got over the fact Nick wouldn't care about our 'song,' I decided to make it all about me. I would pick a song which held a special memory.

I danced with Nick every day before his nap. It started out with my cradling him. When he got older and was sitting up, I would carry him and hold his leg like it was an arm and dance around the house. When he started walking, we would twirl and swing. We danced to whatever I was in the mood for that day, Earth, Wind & Fire, Barry White, Motown, but nine times out of 10, it was Frank Sinatra.

When Nick was a toddler, we went to Florida with our friends John and Peggy. They also had a toddler, their daughter Megan. Peggy was the perfect mother. She fed her kids organic food. I was like here's a French fry. She breast-fed; I bottle-fed. My kids were trained by the microwave bell, kind of like Pavlov's dog. The bell would ring when the bottle was ready, the child would stop crying. I will admit there were times of desperation when to stop the crying I would ring the microwave bell. Desperate times beget desperate measures people. *Don't judge.*

One day, Peggy was playing a cassette tape (yes, that's how long ago it was) of children's songs and Megan was singing along and dancing. I glanced over at Nick, and he was looking at her like she was from another planet. And then it dawned on me: I'm a terrible mother.

I never played children's songs. Nick listened to the music I liked. Note to self: Be a better mom and start playing children's songs.

Fast forward and we're making dinner. While we're preparing, we put in our cassette tape of Frank Sinatra. We're chopping away and listening to old blue eyes when I look over and there is Nick in his glory. He's standing by the coffee table dancing and crooning away to Frank Sinatra. So, because of that memory of a chubby, curly-haired, sausage-hand toddler who couldn't sing a children's song (*because I sucked as a mother*) but could loudly and proudly croon to Frank Sinatra; we danced our mother/son dance to the first song he ever sang—Frank Sinatra's *The Lady is a Tramp*.

> ***So there's this boy, he kind of stole my heart.***
> ***He calls me mom.***
> —Unknown

Really, Insurance?
August 20th

After the first round of chemo, I found I needed the anti-nausea meds more right after an infusion. I was on a two-week cycle with the A/C. The nausea wore off at the end of the cycle. I took the meds religiously during the tough days. I even set my alarm and would take them in the middle of the night, so I didn't wake up sick. I also took a stool softener and, no, we're not going there.

Done with my first cycle and going in for another treatment, I called to have my script refilled. I only had a few pills left and wanted to be prepared for my next round of chemo. My pharmacy informed me my insurance wouldn't cover my script. When I asked why, I was told I was only allowed to have 30 pills every 30 days. Are you kidding me? I was taking four pills a day for the first week to fight the nausea. Those pills were saving me. I really needed them.

I called my insurance. What I really wanted to do was speak to the yahoo who made that edict. I wanted to ask them if they had ever experienced chemo and its side effects. I'm sure they hadn't. No one who experiences this would ever withhold medication from those in treatment. I pled my case with the girl on the other end. She overrode the order, and my script was sent to the pharmacy. All was right in my drug world.

When it was time for my third round of A/C, I thought my script nightmare was over, but it wasn't the case. I was turned down again as it was only two weeks later. I called and was told I could ask for a review. I filed for a review but wouldn't get an answer for three weeks. I could get the prescription but had to pay for it. Three hundred and fifty dollars later, I had my script.

My final round of A/C is coming up. The next round of Taxol is not supposed to make me nauseous. I just need one more script to get me through. I'm once again turned down. I'm angry and in tears. My insurance company is willing to fork out thousands of dollars for chemo but will not allow me to have more than 30 pills to treat the side effects from the chemo. *Really?*

There are some pills left from the last script as I've rationed in case I couldn't get more. Thank God for my oncology nurse who goes to battle for me. She gets both the pharmacy and Blue Cross on the phone. They go round and round and finally Blue Cross relents and gives me 20 pills, not 30 but 20, and only if the pharmacist will vouch for me. *Seriously?* Beggars can't be choosy, and I gladly take what I can get. I will never understand insurance companies—EVER!

On a final note, I received a letter from my insurance two weeks **after** I finished my A/C rounds of chemo. After reviewing my case, it was deemed the script for 30 pills a month was to remain. Reason: The diagnosis didn't justify the need for more medication. *I have no words.*

> ***Life is unfair. And it's not fair that life is unfair.***
> —Edward Abbey

At a Loss
September 4th

Four rounds of A/C are completed. *Whoop! Whoop!* I've gotten through the roughest part of the chemo and started the next round. So, what's the problem? I'm at a loss right now trying to get motivated for this next round and I find I'm slumping.

These past weeks have been a whirlwind. We had the rehearsal dinner on Friday, wedding on Saturday, a brunch on Sunday, moved Riley back to college on Monday, moved Bob's mother out of her condo on Tuesday and then my last A/C chemo on Wednesday. My aunt died on Thursday, and I had a family funeral the following Sunday. Can you say whirlwind?

My doctors tell me I should be a poster child for how to go through chemo. By focusing on exercise, eating well (when I had an appetite), vitamins, and keeping a cheerful outlook, I made it look easy. But it was still challenging.

My first two treatments of A/C were easy in the grand scheme of things. The third treatment took away my sense of taste. I expected to feel the same with the last A/C as I had with the first three.

Unfortunately, the last treatment really knocked me for a loop. I was extremely fatigued, and so nauseous, I laid in bed the entire day the following Tuesday hoping to sleep it away. Drinking water was difficult. I began experiencing leg cramps from being so dehydrated. The way I felt physically was affecting me mentally. I was in a deep dive. I felt like I was failing and was so disappointed in myself.

While wallowing, I think how cancer reminds me every day it's a part of my life. I look in the mirror and see a scarred chest with no breast. I see my bald head. My eyelashes are thinning, as are my eyebrows. For the first time in my life, I'm using an eyebrow pencil and, for someone who doesn't 'do' makeup, it's challenging.

I threw out all my bras the other day. I will not be able to wear a regular bra for at least a year. (*Thinking out loud, I should have had a party and burned them.*) I've bought mastectomy bras and bathing suits.

Whenever I wear either, I insert a prosthesis, then I'm constantly making sure my breasts look even. When I finish with my makeup, I put on a wig before I leave the house. **Daily** reminders.

I'm tired of doing this! Tired of being mentally challenged; of not having a sense of taste, of crippling nausea. I *want* to feel normal again, instead of always punky. I was in a slump.

I began thinking about how much farther I had to go on this journey. I was so focused on the first three intense treatments I would have, leading up to the wedding, I hadn't thought about what followed. I prepared myself for the sprint but hadn't prepared myself for the marathon. I was overwhelmed and had a really hard time staying positive. All I was doing was crying. I didn't like the space I was in, but I couldn't pull myself out.

I was forgetting to stay in the present moment, partly because in the present moment I didn't feel well. I began focusing on the long journey to come 12 more chemo treatments taking me into the end of November. Once completed, six weeks of radiation begins; there will be more side effects to deal with.

It will be nine months after radiation to let my body heal before reconstruction. Another major surgery and recovery. I was on overload. This journey takes me on many peaks and valleys. I was in the valley, and I would stay there for a while.

> *I've come to realize that real growth of character takes place in the valleys of life.*
> —Dave Dravecky

The Taxol Treatment

Beginning Taxol
September 6th

Today I start my next round of the new chemo, Taxol, just two weeks after the last round of A/C. No rest for the weary. I'm still nauseous and even took an anti-nausea med this morning because I was still feeling queasy, thinking to myself will it ever end?

I've been told Taxol will not take as long to administer and the side effects will not be as drastic. I will stay longer since it's my first time to make sure I handle it well.

Inserting the needle into my port hurt this time and continued to hurt afterward, making me a little apprehensive for the next time. Otherwise, I handled it like a pro. I have no idea how my body will handle this chemo; I'm on another journey into the unknown. Trust the process and just flow, Carey.

> *You don't need to see the whole stairway, just take the next step.*
> —Martin Luther King

Turning a Corner
September 13th

I turned a corner today. I had my second treatment of Taxol and did just fine. Tonight, we celebrated Bob's 60th birthday with an impromptu pub crawl in Detroit.

It was pure joy being with my family celebrating wonderful Bob. I had chemo, but it didn't keep me from having fun. And that's what turned it for me. I realized I was letting chemo take over my life. I will *have* my weekly chemo, but it's only one morning a week. The rest of the week is for me to enjoy living.

It seems when I'm down in the valley I need to remind myself I'm healing, that's all. It's all a part of the journey. Yes, I will continue to have my daily reminders. I'll still have chemo treatments and all the side effects. Eventually there will be radiation and reconstruction. But ultimately, I **am** living my life while treating cancer.

I need to acknowledge how far I've come from my diagnosis in April, not how far I still need to go. I *am* growing and learning from this. I *will* be here to experience family moments. So even though it's been rough, I **am** grateful for it.

> *Grateful: Find peace, mindfulness and conscious purpose by being grateful for what you have in life.*
> —Clark A. Katz

My Wigs: Gladys and Fifi
September 14th

I find myself doing things like I still have my hair. When taking a shower, my hands automatically go right to my head to begin shampooing. Afterwards, I wrap it in a towel then realize I don't need it as I have no hair to dry. I've finally stopped reaching for my curling iron and hairbrush when getting ready. Several times a day I try to put my hair behind my ears. Small habits that bring me daily reminders.

There are times I forget, then I walk by a mirror and *whoa, who is that bald woman looking back at me?* The other day I left my house, got into my car, and began driving down the street before I realized I forgot to put my wig on. I don't think I've ever turned my car around that fast before.

I will be 'hairless' for a while. When I say no hair—I mean no hair anywhere (and, no, I'm not going there). I'm even losing the hairs in my nose! *Seriously?*

There are some positives. I no longer have to shave my legs. I don't have to pluck my eyebrows (barely hanging on to them). No more pesky chin hairs. Yes, I said chin hairs. Thank you, menopause. I never have a bad hair day. *See, there is a silver lining.*

When I was diagnosed, I started buying hats and scarves to prepare for the inevitable. Here's a revelation: I looked much better in them when I had actual hair. Without it, not so much. I look like a bald woman in a hat.

I decided wearing a wig would work best for me. I put a lot of pressure on my wigs. After all, they were my first line of defense in managing my changed appearance. I wanted people to look at me and say, "That's a wig?" One day someone told me how she loved my new haircut. (*Yep, that says a lot about my original hair.*)

I've got a tight bond with my wigs; they are my steadfast companions in my journey with the Big "C". They make me look and feel like I don't have cancer. They are doing a great job.

I've named them Gladys and Fifi. I had originally thought they would be named something more sophisticated and glamorous. Monique, Coco, Elisabetta, so many possibilities. But alas, they named themselves. Neither would take no for an answer.

Gladys popped into my head and just wouldn't leave. So, Gladys it is. She's the wig I wear 99% of the time. She looks the most like my original style only better. I finally looked up the meaning of Gladys and besides being a derivative of a flower, it also means royalty or princess. That pretty much sums up my Gladys. She has the traits of a royal. She is loyal, steadfast, and regal.

Fifi, on the other hand, has a totally different vibe. I originally named her Coco, but Fifi seemed to push her way in. She's short, sassy and a little poufy. I wear her when I'm taking a walk on the wild side. Both ladies are serving me well.

When cancer tries to strip you down and steal your dignity, there are little things that can bring you up. My wigs do that for me. My bald head is a beacon that shouts, *"Look she has cancer!"* Gladys and Fifi give me a chance to forget about it for a while and just be Carey. They give me confidence on days when I'm feeling insecure. A wig may seem insignificant in the grand scheme of cancer treatment but being able to feel somewhat normal is priceless. To Gladys and Fifi—you have my immense gratitude for helping me navigate this journey.

> ***Thank you for being my ray of sunshine even on the darkest days.***
> —Unknown

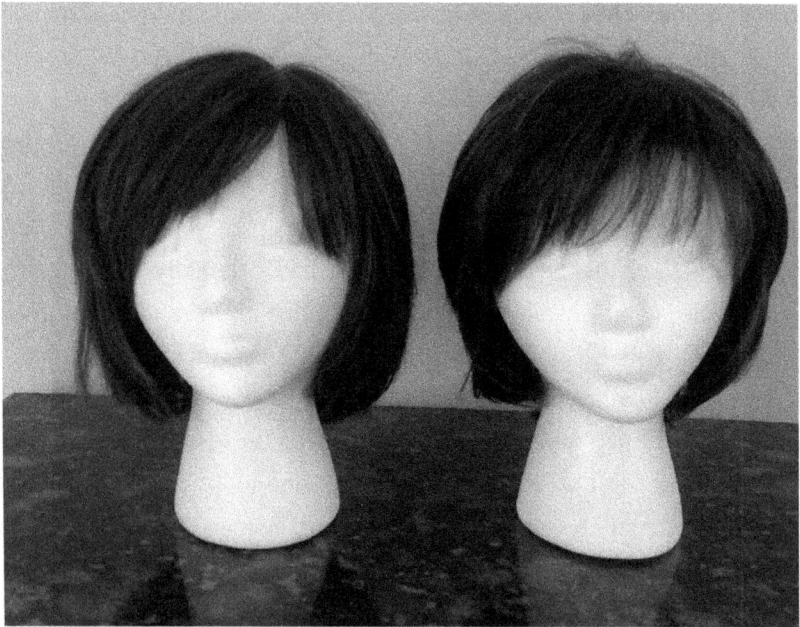

It's All in the Nose
September 16th

When having chemotherapy, I thought I understood where I would lose my hair: basically everywhere. It never entered my mind it would be in my nose! Geez, talk about adding insult to injury. I'm bald, so I wear a wig. I now have to put on my eyebrows. (I feel like Norma Desmond—*"Alright, Mr. DeMille, I'm ready for my closeup."*)

I can count how many eyelashes I have and now with no nose hairs I constantly have a runny nose. At night when I sleep, my nose has no moisture, so I wake up every morning with a bloody nose—yep, these are the good times. Another side effect of treating cancer I certainly didn't see coming.

When my chemo ends, I'm told my hair will begin to grow back. Guess where I hope it grows first? I will forever live in gratitude for those little hairs and will never take them for granted again. Long live nose hairs!

> *We sometimes underestimate the influence of little things.*
> —Charles W. Chestnutt

Desperate Times, Desperate Measures
September 20th

Most of my eyebrows and eyelashes are gone. The ESS I used obviously didn't work. I look in the mirror and try to use makeup to make it appear like I still have them. I feel like a bald man who does the comb-over.

Today, I've hit a new low, people. I'm putting on my makeup as I'm going to a luncheon with my friend, Laurie, and find myself putting mascara on two eyelashes. Yes, I said TWO eyelashes. Like applying mascara on those two piddly eyelashes is going to make a difference. *Really, Carey. OMG, can you say desperate?*

> *Desperate people do desperate things.*
> —Michael Brooks

Thoughts on a Rainy Day
September 27th

It's a rainy, gloomy day and it's almost time for my weekly trip to the infusion center. I'm leaving soon. I'll put numbing cream on my port in a half an hour to prepare the site for the needle insertion. I've packed my bag of goodies (mints, Kindle, warm socks, and bottled water) to take with me. This will be chemo No. 10. I'm receiving the 'easier' chemo now. Today will be my sixth treatment of Taxol, which means I'm halfway through.

Has it been easy? That's a tough question to answer. I've never done it before, so I have nothing to compare. I haven't had to be hospitalized, no fevers. I haven't thrown up or lost weight. *I've gained weight, dammit.* I've maintained my exercise schedule. My blood count numbers have been fine, so I haven't had to reschedule my treatments.

They tell me I've handled the side effects from both chemo treatments extremely well; so well my steroid and Benadryl dosages have been halved. On a good note: I lost five pounds when that happened—*Whoo-hoo.* Yes, going through cancer treatment and still obsessing about weight. Some things never change.

There are days I'm exhausted or as I say to Bob, *"I'm out of power, Luke."* Those are the days when I rest and relax. I won't lie to you and say it's all sunshine and roses because it's not. You do what you need to do to get through—that's all. On the days I'm down, I work hard to realize how far I've come on this journey and the hard times (mastectomy and A/C chemo) are behind me, reminding myself I've chosen this path and all that comes with it.

I try to stay in gratitude for all it has given me and will continue to give me. Love, healing, hope. *Love* I feel from my family and friends, *healing* myself both physically and mentally, and *hope* because of this journey, I will have a future.

I have so much to be thankful for. It may be a gloomy day today, but I only feel sunshine. Bring on Chemo No. 10!

Every storm runs out of rain.
—Maya Angelou

Like a Baby's Behind
October 24th

Another side effect of chemo: **soft skin**. I have never had such smooth skin in my life. Seriously, my skin feels like a baby's behind everywhere. I normally need to moisturize several times a day to hydrate. Not with chemo. Silky smooth. Even Bob has commented on how soft my skin is. So, there you have it—in all the serious side effects from chemo, I've found another positive.

> *Positivity isn't standing in the rain and saying it's not raining. It's about finding a silver lining in the clouds.*
> —Louise Myers

'Senior' Moment
October 26th

I got asked if I was a 'senior' today. I was on my way to my oncology appointment and stopped at Einstein's for a bagel. As I was paying, the cashier smiled and said, "Are you a senior?" I looked at her perplexed and to be honest I was starting to turn my head to look behind me at what I was sure was the real person she was speaking to when I quickly realized that person was me!

My immediate thought was "I look like a senior?" Followed by "OMG, I **am** a senior! When did I become that old?" I obviously don't think I'm a senior. I'm just going to be sixty for God's sake but in my mind I'm much younger.

While contemplating that reality and still not answering, the cashier then said the dreaded word—'Mam?' Not a Miss but a 'Mam!' I've officially turned the corner. OMG! I'm a 'Senior' and a 'Mam!' That sealed it—I now felt old.

Coming out of my shock—I sucked it up, faced reality and responded, "Yes, I am a senior." After admitting to this millennial that

I am old in her eyes; I thought about it for a minute and followed up with "And happy to be one."

You see, I realized in that moment, that even though I'm older, I'm grateful to be a 'Senior.' I'm happy that I'm soon to be 60 and have more years on the horizon. Do I feel like a senior citizen? No. Do I act like a senior citizen? Nope. Do I look like a senior citizen? Hope not. But the reality is that I am, and I embrace it in gratitude.

So, I got my $2.00 senior discount and left smiling. Maybe being a senior has its advantages? Now let's find another word for Mam...

On a side note, when I was at the oncologist, the nurse was going through a list of questions and casually asked, "Are you pregnant?" I looked at her and shouted, *"I'm a senior."* Amazing how I had no problem admitting it then.

> *Know that you are the perfect age. Each year is special and precious, for you shall only live it once. Be comfortable with growing older.*
> —Louise Hay

Singing Bowls
October 27th

In conjunction with traditional medical treatment, I was using various treatments offered by Integrative Medicine. My friend, Mixie, was using singing bowls for meditation and vibrational therapy. She offered to have a session with me. "Just tell me where and when and I'm there," I said. Even if we weren't going to have a singing bowl session, I would go just to be in her presence. She gives off the most peaceful energy.

Tibetan or Himalayan singing bowls are known as a "standing bell." They are played either by rubbing a mallet around the rim (as one might play a crystal glass with a finger) or striking the side of the bowl. The two playing methods produce quite distinctive sounds because the bowls are made of bell bronze which is free of impurities. They are used to aid meditation, relaxation, and healing.

In sound healing, or 'sound massage,' the bowls are placed around or on the body during treatment. The practitioner uses the resonance of the harmonic vibrations for balancing and relaxation.

I went to Mixie's today for a session. It turned out to be one of the most magical times I've had in my healing process. She had me lay on her dining room table. (*Thank God, it was sturdy.*) While lying on the table, she surrounds my body with the bowls, even placing one on my stomach. I take deep cleansing breaths, close my eyes, and wait.

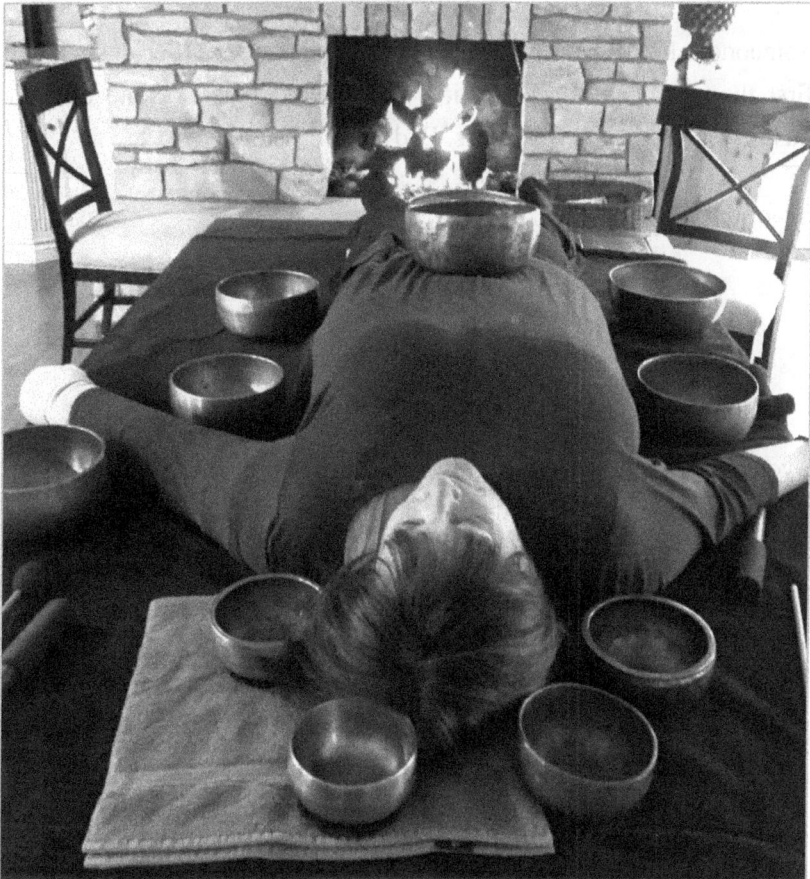

When she begins, I hear beautiful sounds and start to feel the vibrations. My body is absorbing the energy from both. She continued to play for a half an hour. I found myself in such a peaceful state. My meditation went deep. I left feeling reenergized.

Mixie gave me a wonderful gift today, a sense of calm and peace I haven't felt in a long time. Thank you, my friend.

> **To Mixie: When I count my blessings in life, I count you twice.**
> —Carey Cornacchini

Nunya
October 30th

Someone asked me if my husband and I still had sex. (Seriously?) My first thought about that question was 'Nunya' (as in none of your business); but the answer is yes. End of discussion.

> **Hey, I found your nose, it was in my business.**
> —Unknown

Never a Dull Moment
November 4th

I voted today. In the past, it's always been a non-event. At my precinct, there is never a line and if there is, it's minimal. Bob and I head over at 11:00 a.m. Per usual, there is no wait. Bob heads to his cubby and I head to mine, a man in between us.

I set my umbrella down and open my ballot. As I'm reaching for the pen, I feel a snap and it happens. My bra comes undone, and my prosthetic shoots out to the left. Think slingshot—get the picture? Had I not had quick reflexes and slammed my arms to my side, I'm sure the weight and the propulsion of my prosthetic would have killed the man next to me.

I just began the process of voting! Now what? I couldn't stop and snap it shut. Seriously? Can you imagine me asking the voting volunteer, "Excuse me? Could you assist me with something?" Bob was too far away to help and besides we were out in the open.

I looked around, no one knew what had happened but me, so I did what I needed to do. I brought my arms up, holding them tightly to my chest, pressing the prosthetic against my side and voted. It got a little tricky when I had to feed my ballot into the machine. I felt like a T-rex, but I muscled through. Nothing was stopping me from voting, not even a shooting prosthetic.

Today I did my civic duty and once again breast cancer gave me something to laugh about. Breast cancer—never a dull moment!

> *If there was a novel on my life, it would be called never a dull moment.*
> —Maqui688

Just my Luck...
November 8th

Who knew a hurricane would affect me? Today, Donna, my oncology nurse will be administering my chemo meds. She recently switched jobs to the infusion center. It's always nice to see a familiar face. When I sat down, she asked if they had explained to me about the saline shortage. Um, no. A saline shortage?

She proceeds to tell us the factory that supplies the small bags for the saline in Puerto Rico was destroyed during Hurricane Irma; which means the patients who use the small bags of saline are not receiving them. They are estimating it may take a year to get the bags for the saline. *A year?*

When administering the premeds and chemo, an 8 oz. bag of saline is injected through my port. The saline dilutes the drugs being administered and helps hydrate. When she tells us this, I'm not worried as I think the saline was more for hydration than dilution. I would be wrong on that and would find out very quickly the hard way.

Donna is fast when administering my premeds. They're flying into my port. The last one she administers before the actual chemo is

Decadron. At this point, I've assumed my usual position. I've got my warm blankets; my feet are up, and my head is resting comfortably.

We're discussing our families and the upcoming Thanksgiving holiday when she begins to administer the Decadron. *Whoa, Nellie!* My lower back and groin area begin to **severely** itch and burn. I bring my La-Z-Boy to a sitting position and say, "Something is seriously wrong." Donna calmly says you need more saline to dilute it. She administers a syringe of saline, and it goes away. Who knew a little bit of saltwater could do so much good?

The rest of the appointment goes smoothly. I'm now very apprehensive for my next appointment and am hoping by next week the hospital has come up with a plan B.

> ***Plan B. You've always got to have a plan B.***
> —Sylvester Stallone

Radiation Education
November 14th

I made an appointment with the radiation oncologist toward the end of my chemo treatments. I've decided to have Dr. Chen handle my radiation again. I trust him. Trust is important when you're tangling with the Big "C". Having someone you know will give you great care provides peace of mind.

We arrive at the cancer center and when I check in, I'm given a gray key card with my name and patient ID number. I will scan this for entry at each visit.

The first thing I notice when I walk into the office—**no** scale. Six years ago, the scale was right next to the front door. You walked in and weighed yourself, in front of the world. *Yep, good times.*

Bob and I are taken into the examining room where the scale is waiting for me. No evading it, though I was pleased it's located here. Weight and blood pressure taken and as I'm finishing up the mountains of paperwork, the resident walks in. We discuss my medical history, current status, and treatment options.

He walks us through the process and what I can expect from treatment. Because I'm Stage 3, it is highly recommended I have the radiation. It will increase my odds of survival. Side effects include fatigue and possible skin irritation. Information given, he leaves, and we wait for Dr. Chen. He is a kind soul who is extremely dedicated to his work. Work he does extremely well.

We have a kinship since his parents used to live four houses down from us. He knows several of my neighbors. He comes in and after the usual greetings, I ask, "What happened buddy? I did your clinical trial and here I am six years later. I don't think it worked too well." I was joking, thinking it was a great ice breaker. But Dr. Chen responded seriously, "The protocol used last time was the right treatment for your diagnosis—DCIS." (I honestly didn't want to offend him; I was just trying to lighten the mood.)

I tell him they found one milliliter of invasive lobular cancer when they tested the margins. Dr. Chen spends several minutes going through my records and sees that I did indeed have it. He was amazed my surgeon found it. He goes on to explain:

1) What probably happened was there was a stray cell, not in an area where the margins were previously tested, which had been growing for the last six years.

2) Invasive lobular cancer is not detectable by mammograms. I've said this before, but it needs repeating: *Invasive lobular cancer is not detected on mammograms*. My mammogram showed calcification, and, because of that, I had a biopsy. The biopsy identified the invasive lobular cancer.

3) In addition, I had a tumor along with cancer in my skin. In three places—*it was in three places*. It was like my left breast was exploding with cancer.

I'm looking for some good news; where's the silver lining? And I finally get it. He goes on to explain since I did the clinical trial the first time and the treatment went directly to the affected cancerous area, I qualified for radiation. In other words, if I had had traditional radiation the last time, my body would have already had radiation in my chest wall, and I wouldn't have qualified for any radiation. I think, "Everything happens in its own time." I am very lucky.

I ask if I qualify for proton therapy. It's a relatively new therapy that is less invasive. The radiation is administered to an exact pinpointed area instead of the entire breast. My cancer was located in my left breast, so I have concerns about being radiated too close to my heart. If I have a choice, I want the proton therapy. Dr. Chen says we'll discuss how I'll be evaluated when I'm being fitted for radiation. Which led me to my next question—"Fitted?"

To keep my upper body centered during radiation, my head, neck, and upper arms will lay in my personal mold. During the fitting, I will lay on a warm form which will shape to my body. This form is used for every treatment.

I'll be tattooed (not happy) on three different points. The tattoos are used to align my body with the machine. Since I will be radiated on my left side, they will need to see where my heart sits in my chest wall. *Can't wait for this to happen—not.*

I will be seeing Dr. Chen once a week during treatment. He walks us over to the appointment center; gives me a hug and says I'll see you soon. Appointment made: December 18th is the fitting.

We then meet with Bev the radiation nurse. I immediately like her energy. She tells me she had been through radiation for cancer years ago. I like hearing that as she truly understands what I will go through. She puts me at ease. She has us watch an informational video. It's about five minutes long and explains the procedure along with the possible side effects.

Video done; Bev comes back to answer any more questions. I want to know if my skin will burn. She tells me it's a possibility. They will monitor my skin for any concerns. If there is damage, astringents and lotions could help. She reminds me this is temporary. I chuckle to myself; I seem to always need to get *that* reminder. She gives me a packet of information and we're good to go. I swear with all the information I have received I could start a library.

We leave the office and I'm quiet on the way home, thinking about my diagnosis. I usually ignore it. Logically, I know I've had cancer, and it was advanced, but I don't think about the details and today I figured out why. Details drag me down. They can sound so dire. Doom and gloom. If I dwell on it, it's like I'm saying, "Hey, fear, come on in." I stay in a dark place for a while, thinking about the severity of my diagnosis. I eventually remind myself I was estrogen positive, which is a good thing, medical advances have come a long way and I've been given a great success rate. It's a struggle at times to get back to center, but I always get back there and for that I'm thankful. On to the fitting.

> *Take a deep breath, pick yourself up, dust yourself off, and start all over again.*
> —Frank Sinatra

Let's Try This Again...
November 15th

We arrive today and low and behold, I get Anna, my very first chemo nurse. Since I'm extremely apprehensive about the burning I felt last time, I'm glad I have a familiar face administering the chemo today.

While walking back, I run into Donna, she confirms it was the Decadron which caused my pain. I tell Anna about my fears being the big baby that I am. She said she would dilute the Decadron in saline before she administers it and follow up with a syringe of just saline. She would also administer it very slowly. Not the full bag of saline but hopefully it will work. I feel a little bit better. Still apprehensive, but there's a plan.

She begins with the Pepcid, and it goes well. Unbeknownst to me, she administers the Decadron next. She does this very, very slowly. I feel nothing. It works! I'm pain free. My anxiety has left my body. She follows with the Benadryl. My head gets my usual fog, but other than that it was uneventful. I know I can survive the premeds and chemo without my eight-ounce bag of saline. Life just got back on kilter.

> *Those that are resilient can more quickly regain their equilibrium and spring back when they are thrown off kilter with the storms in life.*
> —Mary Buchan

One Last Poke!
November 20th

I had my last poke today. As part of the chemo process, I've had to have a blood test within three days of each chemo treatment to determine whether my blood is at the right levels. I have been lucky it's always come back fine and haven't had to reschedule any of my treatments.

I have driven to the hospital every Monday to get my blood work. Every other week for the first four A/C chemo treatments, then once a week for my 12 Taxol treatments. That's sixteen pokes.

Sixteen times where I've driven, parked, walked in and waved to the security guard. Presented my blue card and repeated my name and birthdate. Sat in the waiting room holding my card with a letter on it. (Since I'm a regular, I get a letter not a number—letters get called sooner.) Waiting in my chair for a tech (or vampire as they refer to themselves) to draw my blood; once again repeating my name and birthdate; pushing up my sleeve, making a fist while my arm is being tied off. Feeling the poke and watching while two vials are filled with my blood, then receiving a bandage on my new wound (hoping it doesn't bruise.) Finally, driving home, keeping my fingers crossed my blood work will be fine.

My last blood draw is done. It's completed. I've jumped over another hurdle. It seems this journey has been about hurdles. Keeping myself focused to jump another one. So today, I've jumped the last one which will take me to the finish line, and it feels just fantastic!

> *Hurdles are always in life; it all depends on how you take it—*
> *as a hurdle or as a path to move ahead.*
> —Rashik Rastogi

One of the Best Days Ever!
November 22nd

I have my last chemo today. Let me write that appropriately: I HAVE MY LAST CHEMO TODAY! It's finally here. When I began my chemo journey on July 12th, Nov. 22nd seemed light years away. Fear was so prevalent during my first treatment. My mind was in overdrive worrying about the unknowns. I was not doing well at staying present as I kept wondering how I was going to survive this.

I find myself overcome with so many emotions today. I woke up crying. Part of me is sad I had to take this journey. I mourn for the old me. The person who had hair, a body that wasn't cut and scarred; the carefree version who thought I was done with cancer six years ago. I also mourn for the journey yet to come.

Eventually those sad tears turned to joy realizing how far I **have** come. How much I've accomplished. The fears I started with are long gone. I've learned apprehension is worse than reality. I've adjusted to not having hair and I don't cringe anymore when I look at my body in the mirror. Always reminding myself this is what healing looks like and it's temporary.

I was watching television last night and a commercial came on for Neulasta (a drug given to help build your immune system after intense chemo). Bob looked over and tears were streaming down my face. He asked me what was wrong, and I told him, "I can't believe I went through this." This has been one of the most challenging things I've ever had to experience. I look back on the days when I would say to

Bob, "I'm so tired of feeling nauseous and exhausted. I can't wait to feel good again." And I'm almost there.

When I have my last chemo today, I'll be tired and slightly nauseous. My sense of taste will still be gone, but it's all temporary. In the next few weeks, I'm hoping to get some of my old self back. How *great* will that be? I'm lucky enough to have the month of December off before I begin my next phase of treatment and I'm incredibly thankful for it. What a holiday it will be for my family. But right now, I can't wait to start my day!

> **Sometimes the bad things that happen in our lives put us directly on the path to the best things that will ever happen to us.**
> —Nicole Reed

Ring the Bell
November 22nd

I'm uber excited on the way to the hospital. Bob, Riley, and Anthony are with me today. Nick is flying so he can't join us. We're wearing our pink leis. I've brought my signature 'boob' cake pops to pass out to everyone. *It's a celebration.*

My nurses and aides—where do I start? I knew them before when I volunteered, but during chemo I have gotten to really know each and every one of them. I've learned about their lives and watched their commitment to helping people like me going through a difficult journey. During my visits, they've made me feel comfortable (love my warm blankets), safe and even made me laugh. My chemo treatments were enjoyable because of them. They **are** my angels.

When my infusion was finished, they all came into my room to watch me ring the bell. Having them all there on that last day was perfect. Anna who was the first nurse to administer my chemo held the bell for me to ring. I rang the bell with all my heart. I wanted it to be

loud enough, so the entire world knew I was done. *Completed, Finished.*
I feel like I just climbed Mt. Everest and I was standing at the top.
It was hugs all around. Love for all those who have been with me on
this journey and gratitude that I was given this journey in order to have
a life. *I Did It! Whoop! Whoop!*

> ***The best view comes from the hardest climb.***
> —Unknown

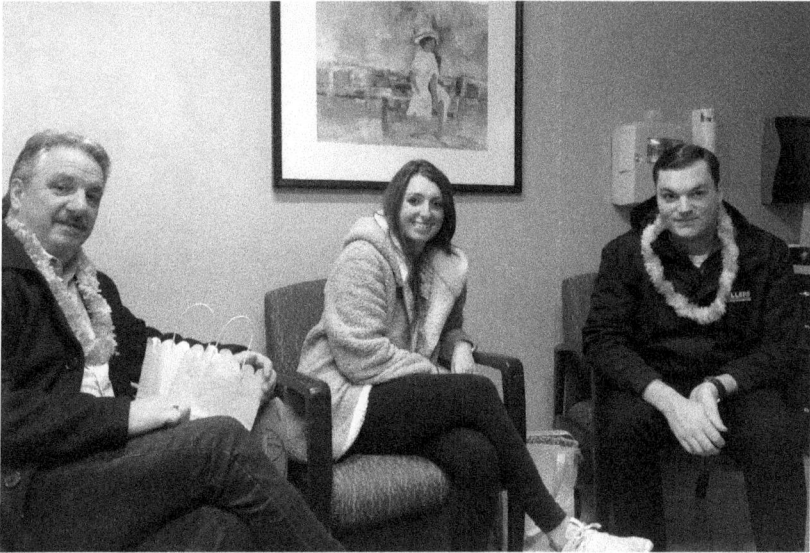

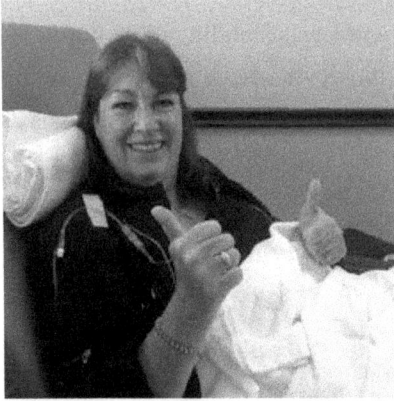
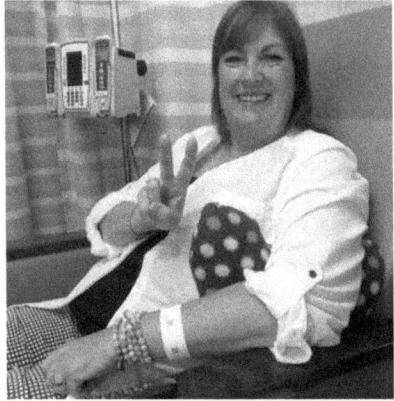
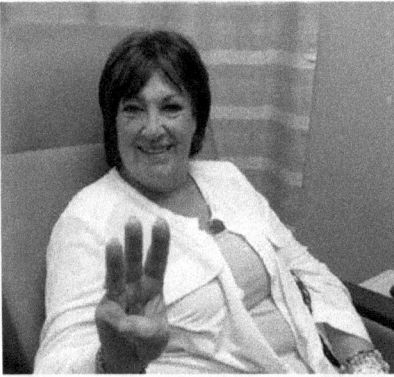
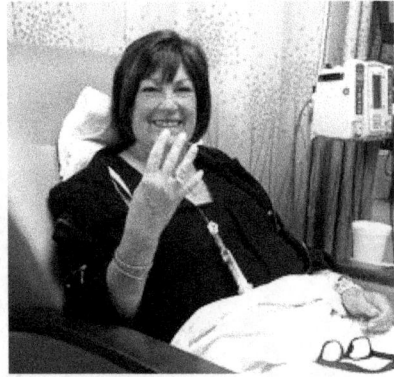
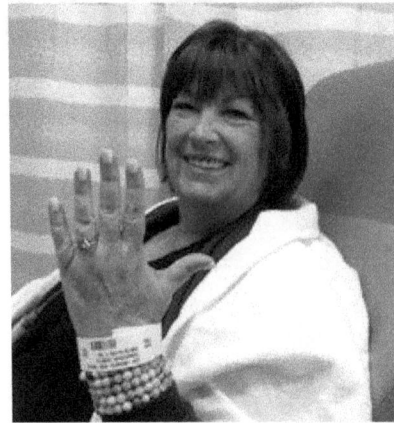
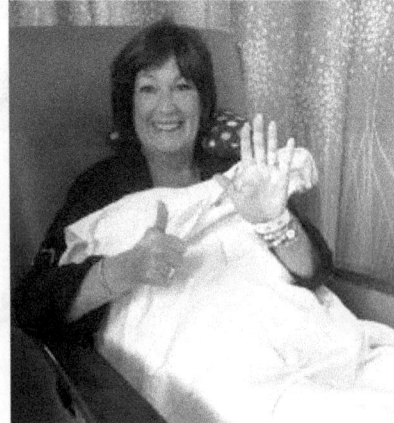

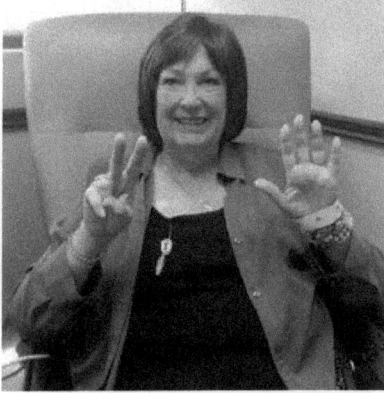

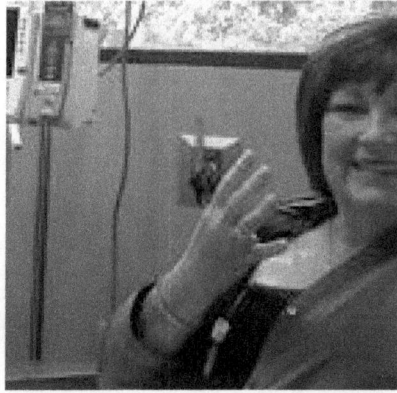

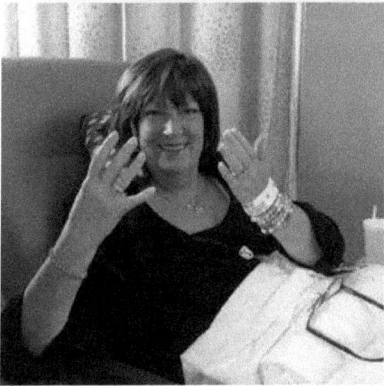

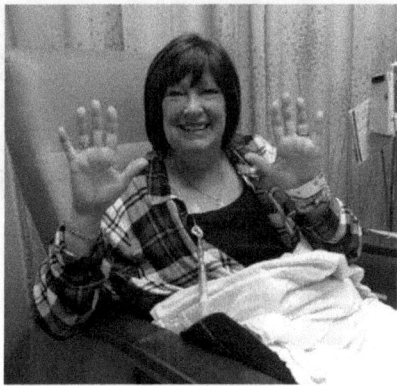

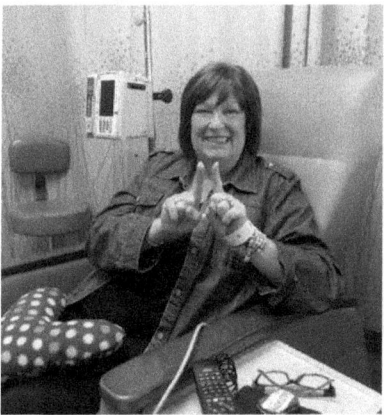

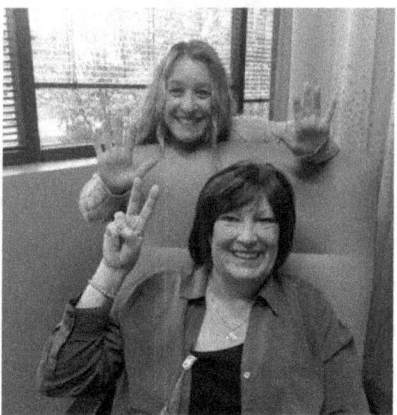

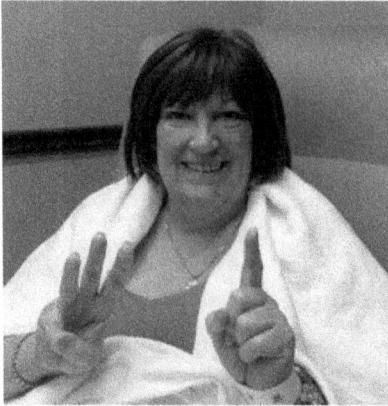

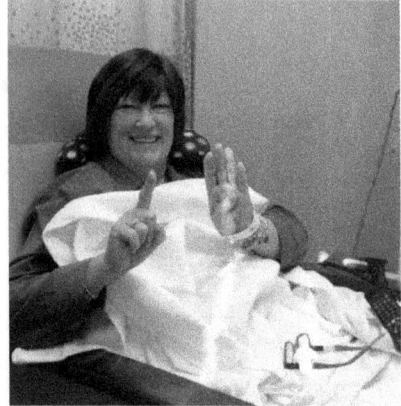

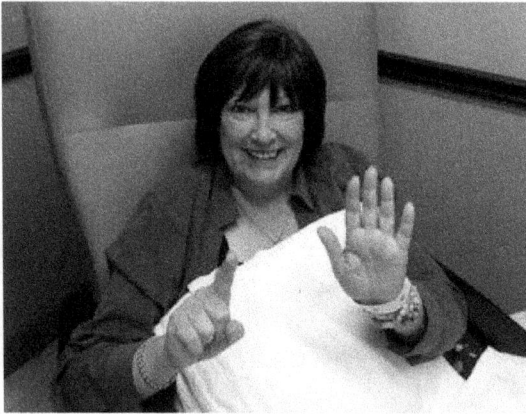

Anthony
November 23rd

Anthony was my only child living at home during my treatments, so he witnessed my journey more than my other two. He saw me on the days when I was exhausted and nauseous, times where frustration and anger were present, He saw it all. I worried about him. He was going to school and working a full-time job. He was busy, his plate was full. He told me later he wanted to be busy as it was hard to watch me go through it.

He didn't verbalize much to me when I would prod (*because that's what mothers do*) making me wonder how he was digesting all of this. But when he did share, it always touched my heart. His postings on

Instagram and Facebook were heartfelt and filled with love. Yesterday, after he witnessed my last chemo, he posted this on Facebook:

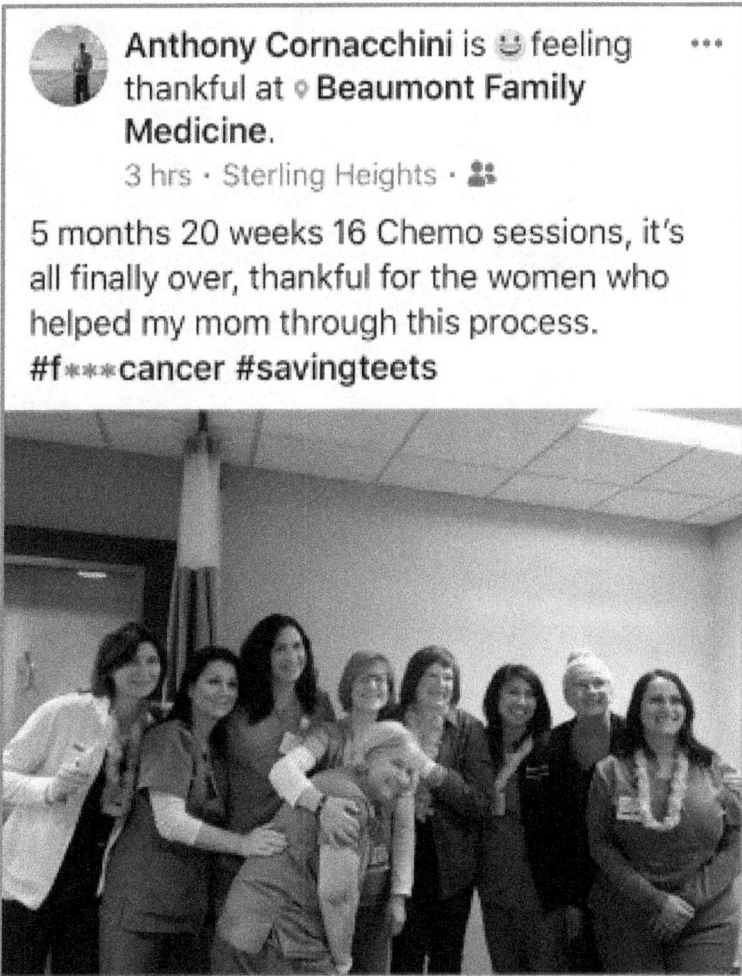

Anthony Cornacchini is ☺ feeling thankful at ⚲ **Beaumont Family Medicine.**

3 hrs · Sterling Heights · 👥

5 months 20 weeks 16 Chemo sessions, it's all finally over, thankful for the women who helped my mom through this process. #f***cancer #savingteets

He once again blew me away with his insight. He cares, he loves and knows gratitude. As a parent, I couldn't be prouder. Thank you, 'Cheek,' for choosing me as your mother.

> *Happiness is when you realize your children have turned out to be good people.*
> —Unknown

Pre-Radiation

Is That a Hair?
December 15th

One of the many things I was looking forward to when I ended chemo treatments was having hair again. Not only hair on my head, but what I really wanted were eyebrows and eyelashes. Every day there was a thorough examination in the magnified mirror to see if there was an eyelash or eyebrow forming. Fingers were crossed daily hoping to see some progress.

It finally happened this morning. Were my eyes deceiving me? Was that a hair I was seeing? It was! I had a hair! Notice I said "a" hair. *One.* I had *one* hair. While I was pleased my body was producing hair, I was not thrilled with its location.

You see, I finally get a hair and it's on my chin. Yep, my chin. Wait, it gets better. It's white. *OMG Really?* Is this the universe's idea of a cruel joke? I have a white chin hair? It was bad enough having chin hair when it was black, but white?

I quickly grab the tweezers and remove the offending hair. Laughing to myself afterwards, I thought just my luck—I finally get hair, it's on my chin and it's *white*. Story of my life. Quickly getting over my indignance, I smile. My body made a hair albeit not where I wanted it, but it made a hair. I got to do something normal today. I plucked a pesky chin hair. The road back to normalcy is beginning. *Whoop! Whoop!*

> *Normalcy to me is enjoying the simple things in life.*
> —Atticus Shaffer

Grrr! You're So Brave
December 17th

Someone said to me today: "You're so brave—your courage is unbelievable." I've heard those words from many people and bristle every time I hear it. I don't consider what I'm doing brave *or* courageous. I'm just navigating my way through. I've been thrust into a situation that I have no control over and I'm figuring it out just like everyone else.

People have told me, "I could never handle it as well as you have." How do you know? I believe each of us has a reserve of strength we don't know we possess. None of us knows how we will handle any situation until we're in it. I'm in it and doing the best I can. That's all. I take each day as it comes. Some days are better than others. But the bottom line is I get to **have** days. When you're faced with a diagnosis of Stage 3 cancer, you appreciate the days no matter what they bring. I'm grateful to have them.

Life can be frightening, but it can also be beautiful. Why waste my time dwelling on the negative? When I get up every morning, my first thought is gratitude. I'm grateful for another day. I then have a choice to make—be happy or be sad. Simple, really. I can decide what type of day I'll have.

This quote from Wayne Dyer sums it up perfectly for me:

With everything that has happened to you, you can either feel sorry for yourself, or treat what has happened as a gift. Everything is either an opportunity to grow, or an obstacle to keep you from growing. You get to choose.

I choose to look at my journey with the Big "C" as a gift. It has given me an opportunity to grow and learn, to experience love and care, to really love myself and to understand, once again, how precious life is.

There's another quote I love from Anne Dennish: *"When you replace 'why is this happening to me' with 'What is this trying to teach me?' everything shifts."*

It does shift. I don't want to give energy to being a victim. I look at everything that has happened to me as a learning opportunity. Another footstep in my path of life. All my life experiences, even those which frustrate me, give me lessons, and contribute to my growth. I am who I am today because of those experiences and I'm grateful.

> **Above all, be the heroine in your life, not the victim.**
> —Nora Ephron

The Fitting
December 18th

Today I have an appointment to have a fitting for the form which will be used in my radiation treatments. One more thing to prepare me for the next step.

I want to go alone so I can get the lay of the land. After all, I'll be driving this route every day for the next six weeks. I arrive and park in patient parking. Another bonus: The spots are closer. I walk down the flight of stairs and swipe my barcoded patient card. Checked in, changed into the requisite hospital gown, and taken to the imaging room. I recognize this room; I've been here before. This was the machine which found the faulty Contura from my first dance. Something familiar. I'm more at ease.

I'm greeted by three radiation therapists. They have me lay down arms over my head on a table. I'm moved into the CT tunnel. It covers my upper body. Not too claustrophobic. Several scans are taken. Once this is completed, it's time to make the mold.

They ask me to lay back into a warm mold. Since it's warm, the mold will form quickly. I begin to lay back and hear, "You'll want to remove your wig because the heat could melt it." Come on, I'm laying semi-topless in front of strangers and now I have to take off my wig? I swear there's no dignity with this disease.

I reach up and pull it off. No reaction from anyone. Then I remember this is an everyday occurrence for them. They are not here to judge but to help heal. You can't work in this environment day after day and not

161

be a person of compassion. I have always been treated with the utmost respect and caring. More testament to angels on earth.

Wig off, I lay back into the warm mold. I place my arms above my head. I assume this is how I'll lay for radiation. Once the mold is made, I get my tattoos. Yes, I said tattoos. I ask James, who is giving me the tattoos, if tattooing is part of their curriculum. He smiles and says it was on-the-job training. I've never wanted a tattoo and am not too happy that I'll have three.

I really shouldn't complain; they're just dots. I tell him I'd rather have tiny four-leaf clovers. Could he do that? He laughs. "Stay still and don't jump," he says. Immediately, that tells me this could be painful. *Great.* Deep breath. I tell him to go ahead. I felt a pinch. Then another. I have two dots. One on each side, just above my hips. They will give me a third tattoo on the test run. Preparation complete.

I'm concerned about the timing of my treatment as I want to go away during the holidays. I'm told it will take a few weeks to evaluate all the data to come up with my correct treatment plan. I will get a call in the beginning of the year. Vacation safe, time to just rest and be. It's going to be a joyous Christmas and New Year!

> *Before anything else preparation is the key to success.*
> —Alexander Graham Bell

Pat on the Back
December 20th

When I began my Taxol regime of chemotherapy, I was told the most common side effect could be neuropathy in my fingers and toes. This usually occurs about halfway through the treatments. I was to have 12 treatments, so around Week 6, it might appear.

Week six came and went and no neuropathy. Maybe I would be one of the lucky ones. Alas, as I found with most of the side effects, I was not the exception. When my treatment ended, I had neuropathy in two of my toes and, appropriately, my middle finger. Not so bad. I was told it usually goes away within a few months. In the grand scheme of side effects, this would be a breeze.

As time passed, my neuropathy got worse. It was now in all my fingers and toes. It's like they are perpetually asleep. I find grabbing things difficult. I can't open jars. I'm constantly wiggling my toes to see if there's feeling. Try wrapping Christmas presents when your fingers have neuropathy. I've found a new appreciation for gift bags!

Slowly but surely the feeling started to come back. It took a few months, but now I have full feeling in all my extremities. Once again, my body had to endure extreme medication to heal. I'm pretty proud of her and all she has gone through. She surprised me on how well she bounced back. Who knew?

I've finished the first part of my treatment and worked my way through all the side effects. The worst is over, and I did it. I'm giving myself a pat on the back. Job well done, Carey, job well done. Bring on the next phase.

> *I'd like to congratulate myself, and thank myself, and give myself a big pat on the back.*
> —Dee Dee Ramone

A Girl in Any Port
December 22nd

It's been strange having a port in my body, located on the upper right side of my chest right under my skin. A foreign object is in my body and if I lay a certain way or bump against something, I feel it. Once my chemo treatments are done, I want it out immediately. Imagine my disappointment when Dr. Ruark told me she wants to wait at least three weeks to let my body heal from chemo. (That would bring me into December.) Not happy but resigned, my removal is scheduled for December 21st.

Dr. Ruark's office calls me in the beginning of December, the doctor has fallen and broken her elbow. She will be out of commission for at least six months. (*Poor Dr. Ruark.*) My appointment to remove my port is in two weeks. Now what?

After several phone calls and mix-ups, the office is able to set an appointment with the radiology group, December 22nd, only one day later than the original date and before Christmas. *Whoo-hoo!*

I have no apprehension for this surgery. When the port was inserted, I was given twilight sleep and was home and feeling fine later that day. *Easy peasy!*

The hospital calls to get the usual prerequisite information. After confirming the time, I swiftly go through the question portion (once again having to tell my weight ☹—does it ever end?) Instructions are next. Honestly after so many surgeries, I know them by heart. While she's talking, my mind wanders. I tune back in time to hear her say I can have liquids like coffee in the morning. "Excuse me? But I'm not to have anything after midnight due to the anesthesia." She responds, "You aren't having anesthesia. You are having a local."

Remember how I said I'm not worried about the surgery? Well, I've just done a 180. A local? How many shots will it take to numb the area? How deep will they have to go? This does not sound easy peasy, it sounds horrific.

Anxiety level is at an all-time high, I have to wait two weeks for the surgery. You would think by now I would get over my aversion to needles. I never really dreaded them before, but considering the number of times I've been poked, where I've been poked, and the numbing medication that burns like a *itch, yep, I'm apprehensive.

At the hospital, we find a packed waiting room. Name given, seat taken, now the wait. Just what my anxiety needs. *Breathe it out, Princess.* We sit for over an hour before I'm taken back and led into a bay. They tell me I've been squeezed in, hence, the delay. The nurse says the doctor is very methodical. He's a perfectionist and takes his time. Okay, then, the wait will be worth it.

I'm finally wheeled into a tiny room with an operating table. The top half of my body is taped, leaving a square opening where the port resides. Brown disinfectant is smeared over the opening. Petrified would describe me right now. *God, I hate cancer.*

The doctor arrives. He seems like a quiet man, a little on the shy side. Well, he hasn't met me, and I tend to talk when I'm nervous. He's not going to know what hit him.

What I've been dreading begins. I'd like to say the apprehension was worse than the reality, but then I'd be lying. It hurt like *hell*. Usually after the first injection to numb the area, the following injections don't hurt. Not the case here. At one point during another painful injection, I started singing a Christmas song. I bellowed, *"Oh, the weather outside is frightful, but the fire is so delightful . . ."* right into the chorus of *"Let it snow, let it snow, let it snow."*

I have **no** idea where that came from, but it was either sing or scream. The doctor stops with an incredulous look on his face. I'm quite sure he's never heard someone singing during this procedure. I look at him and say, "Any requests?" Laughter was needed right now. Deep breath in, I tell him to continue, taking everything in me to hold still. Finally, numbness begins to set in.

When completely numb, he begins. Time to start interrogating the quiet guy. He's an interventional radiologist. It sounds like a jack-of-trades type of job. Performing surgeries like port insertion and removal are minor aspects of what he does. He also places catheters for dialysis, and instruments to dissolve blood clots and drainage. In addition, he performs biliary intervention in several types of cancer treatments. I get Mr. Shy to talk the entire time. Amazing.

As we're talking, he's busy working. There is no pain (yay!) and after much tugging, the port is removed. The doctor stitches me up and I'm done. *Whew!* The nurse cleans me up as best she can, and I'm wheeled back to the bay area to find there's no room for me.

All I need to do is dress, so I ask if I can change in the bathroom. The bathroom, it is. *Desperate times.* Bob helps me. We're laughing because we're trying not to touch anything, too many germs. We're playing the adult version of the *lava game*. I finally got dressed after much laughing. Back in the wheelchair with home care instructions, we go to the valet. Once again, I'm clamoring into the truck. I swear Bob never brings something easy to get into.

As we head home, he puts his hand on my arm and asks how I'm doing. I can't hold it in any longer. I begin to sob, that was a rough one. It's the first time I've had real pain in a procedure. I am more thankful than ever for my breast surgeon. She always gives her patients twilight sleep for port surgeries. She makes a painful experience stress-free.

Cancer patients undergo many tests and surgeries. We are more than willing to endure a lot for a chance at a longer life. Today's procedure bordered on barbaric. I think of the patients who don't have a doctor to ensure they have a painless port insertion and feel immense sadness that others will experience this. Treating cancer is hard enough, having immense pain during a procedure is unacceptable.

Once home, I collapse in my ever-faithful lazy boy. I'm mentally exhausted. While falling asleep, I think about my day. The procedure was a horrible experience, but it's done. The worst is over. My port is out. That port was my last tie to chemo. No port, no chemo. A *major* milestone accomplished. One step closure to the finish line.

> *Remember to celebrate the milestones as you prepare for the road ahead.*
> —Nelson Mandela

Christmas Letters
December 25th

I started a Christmas tradition with my children when they were younger. I didn't want any presents from them. I asked for a letter. I wanted them to write to me about their year. What they experienced, what they learned and their goals for the coming year. They were in grade school when I started this tradition, so I have a diary of their lives. These letters are one of my most treasured possessions.

Their writing has evolved over the years. I think the first year, I received a card from Anthony it just said, *"Merry Christmas, Anthony."* Not even "Love, Anthony." The next year I got two lines, *"Merry Christmas, I love you, Anthony."* He eventually got the hang of it, and I have gotten some doozies. One of my favorites was when he turned 16. Anthony's life revolved around two things: food and CARS. He couldn't wait to get his license. Sixteen couldn't come fast enough for him; we, on the other hand, could wait a while longer. His Christmas letter when he was 16 went something like this:

> *I turned 16 this year, it's been pretty uneventful, except for the fact that I got my license. I'm not doing too bad driving. I've had two accidents of which you know of one, well I guess you know of the other one now. I brought the street sign home to prove to you it wasn't my fault...*

The letters are the last thing I open. All eyes are on me. Moral dilemma: Do I mention the car accident and watch my calm, at-peace husband, blow a gasket on Christmas or do I save this little tidbit until Dec. 26th? And guess what wins out? I finish reading the letter, hug Anthony and whisper in his ear, "We need to talk later."

Over the years, I've read about their triumphs and tragedies, how they overcame their adversities, what they learned from them. Some years were harder to read than others.

I wasn't sure if I was going to get any letters this year. Nothing had been said. Nick was married now. Would I still get them? There were two letters on the tree on Christmas morning with both kids telling me Nick was bringing his later. I was getting letters. *Whoop! Whoop!*

What I received this year touched my soul. While each wrote about things they had done throughout the year, they also told me how my diagnosis had affected them. Each of them pouring their hearts out, explaining how they coped. How they got strength from each other. They told me what they learned from watching my journey and how much I am loved. They were honest and real about their feelings. Reading about their fear and heartbreak was difficult, but each of them ended their letters with hope for the future.

Cancer doesn't just affect me. It has tentacles which are far-reaching. Every family member is touched by the Big "C", each taking their own journey, trying to navigate their gamut of emotions. They, too, experienced anger, fear, frustration, and helplessness. I think it's harder for those watching to feel joy as easily as I do. It's painful to watch a loved one go through cancer. As Anthony said in his letter: *"I was so frustrated and angry because I couldn't fix it for you."*

Reading their letters and seeing they ended with love and hope made my heart lighter. Cancer came into our lives, once again, and gave us many gifts. We learned, we grew, and we loved. Reading those letters gave me a sense of peace. It showed me we are all on the path of healing.

> **When you have cancer, the whole family and everyone that loves them does too.**
> —Terri Clark

Endless Possibilities!
December 31st

The new year is here. 2018, on to new beginnings. Out with the old, in with the new. How do I feel about the 'old'? Can I even wrap my feelings around my last year?

Every New Year's, I always contemplate what the universe is going to bring me. What life events will I experience? What am I to learn this year? Will I be able to embrace what is brought to me?

Going into 2017 with those thoughts, I never imagined the year ahead of me. It was one of my most memorable and challenging. While it brought fear, grief, pain, and sadness, it also brought humor, love, gratitude, joy, and hope.

We spent New Year's Eve in Bay Harbor near Petoskey (thank you, Laurie). The kids opted to go to a party, while Bob and I opted to stay in the condo and have a quiet New Year's. We turned off all the lights, sat by the fire and opened a bottle of red.

There's something hypnotic about staring at a fire. Meditative in a way. It can bring you in deep quickly. We were both lost in our own worlds while staring at the flames. Talking later, we found we both had the same thought—2017. At one point, we just looked at each other and said, *"What was that?" "Did that really happen?"* We talked about how quickly our lives changed and all we've been through. How we are so grateful for each other. When I think about the last six months of the year and all that has occurred, my mind can hardly catch up.

Again, I'm living proof that "Life can turn on a dime." I was a survivor. Then *boom*. I'm Stage 3. Last year, when thinking about my upcoming 2017, cancer never entered into the picture.

How do I really feel about 2017? Do I wish it away? No. The universe gave it to me. It is part of my path. It's another chapter in my story. Last year, I was physically and mentally challenged beyond anything I'd ever experienced. Cancer and all the baggage it brings with it. Yes, it was awful at times, but when looking back, the positive outweighs the negative. I found strength, hope and humor. How can I not feel it was a good year?

I turn the page with gratitude for 2017 and all it has given me. I'll take what I've learned and look forward to what the universe has in store for me in 2018. Bring on the next phase of treatment. No matter what happens, life is going to give me endless possibilities!

> *Life is filled with endless possibilities.*
> —Lailah Gifty Akita

A Trip of a Lifetime
January 8th

It's the new year and I'm finally seeing a glimpse of the end of the tunnel. I will be done with treatment by the end of February. I want to celebrate the end of this journey. Bob and I decide to take a family trip.

We offer three options to the kids: an Alaskan cruise, Ireland, or Italy. Riley and Nick opt for Ireland, Anthony the cruise. Majority wins out—Ireland it is.

A friend recommends a travel agent from Ireland, Cathal O'Donoghue. (Isn't that the coolest name?) He was everything Irish with the brogue to match. When we began planning our trip, we thought we would rent a van and drive ourselves. My husband and I did this 31 years ago. Our friend who's been to Ireland over 40 times, strongly suggested a driver this time. You won't regret it, he said.

My mind immediately flashed to an image of all six of us driving in a foreign country, on the other side of the road with no idea where we were going. Nope, all I could imagine was another fine Cornacchini family moment with us in the middle of nowhere, reading Gaelic Road signs and the Italian/Irish tempers coming out. That sealed it, we would hire a driver. Cathal helps me plan a trip of a lifetime for the first week in June. We'll have a driver who will show us magical Ireland and take time as a family to celebrate life. *Whoop! Whoop!*

> *Life should not only be lived, it should be celebrated.*
> —Osho

Testing... And a One and a Two
January 11th

I'm at the hospital this morning for a "run-through" prior to my first radiation. I arrive and change into the uniform (those lovely hospital gowns) and am taken to the room where my treatments will take place.

I see a familiar face—James. It seems he'll be with me on the next phase. I'm happy to have a familiar face.

I lay on a table. My legs are placed on a foam box to lift my knees. My feet are strapped together. They're making sure there is no movement. My personal foam mold is at the top of the table with a machine behind it. I lay down into it, arms over my head. Once in place, James places a clip on my nose and places a tube in my mouth. I will be breathing through this tube.

I'm to take in a deep breath. This raises my chest and places my heart away from the radiation. While I'm taking a deep breath, they will cut off my oxygen. I'm given a panic button to hold which will allow me to breathe should I need it. Just the fact that I have to have a panic button makes me leery.

Before they cut off my oxygen, they take their time with me, taking measurements, moving me millimeters at a time. I keep hearing 90.5. I joke it must be my radio station.

I'm finally moved into the correct spot and the test run begins. The minute they clamp my nose, I get claustrophobic. How am I going to do this? They haven't even cut off the oxygen yet.

I immediately begin reciting the Our Father and Hail Mary. *Pray it out, princess.* While praying, I slowly take deep breaths to get used to the tube. Each breath begins to bring calm. I breathe in **gratitude**, pause in **grace**, and release into **grounding**. I end the trial run with a sense of peace. I can do this. It may be a little uncomfortable, but like chemo, it is doable. Onward and upward—radiation, here I come!

> *It is our attitude at the beginning of a difficult task which, more than anything else, will affect its successful outcome.*
> —William James

Really, Universe? (My Life Was Too Dull?)
January 11th—Later in The Day

I guess the universe decided I didn't have enough on my plate. The day started with my trial run for radiation. It goes fine. Arriving at 9:00 and back home by 10:30; stoked! I'm excited this is going to be a cakewalk.

I had made plans to meet my friend Tina at Lifetime. I'm trying to get in the pool as much as I can before Monday when I begin my radiation treatments. Once I begin those, I'm not allowed to swim.

It's the first time I wear a wig to the club. I always wear a cap. The girl at the front desk notices. We speak as I'm walking by. And then it happens. My foot gets caught in uneven carpet/tile and turns. As I'm trying to correct myself, I hear a pop. The pain was excruciating. So how does my body handle it? I start *fainting*. Now I'd like to tell you I looked like a beautiful Victorian lady who just came down with the vapors, you know slowly and elegantly laying down on a chaise. That would be NO.

I'm asked if I'm alright. I respond, "No, I need to sit down." She grabs a chair and sets it right in the front of the spa where everyone walks in. I can't faint in the back of the locker room. No, I get to faint in the front entrance to Lifetime.

As I stagger over to the chair, I plop into it. Nothing dainty here—full-boat PLOP! I barely make it into the chair when it's lights out for me. Someone called a code, and as I was in and out of consciousness I look up and 20 people are staring at me. All employees. Jesus, it looks like the entire staff is here. This is turning out to be a *bad* day.

At one point, I say there are too many of you, go back to work. Still lightheaded, they move me into the spa and out of the center entrance. I'm sitting, my feet are up, and I'm sweating profusely. I've lost all color in my face.

There is a doctor who is working out who asks if she can check me. I'm fine with that. I tell her I'm so hot (which she can obviously tell as I'm dripping). I take off my coat and am still burning up. I tell her I have a wig on, and she tells me to take it off to feel better. OMG, really? Wig off in front of all these people?

The time has come. I either continue to sweat profusely, and feel faint, or take off my wig and feel cooler. I look at the crowd around me and say, "Sorry guys, but I have to do this, get ready for the show." I am coming out. I take it off. I instantly feel cooler. I've just whipped my wig off in front of everyone at Lifetime. I honestly don't care at this point because I'm so hot I just want relief.

I ask my trainer Sherry, who's staying right by my side, if someone could tell my friend Tina, I won't be meeting her in the pool. Tina gets out of the pool and says, "Really Carey, you'll do anything to get out of swimming." She follows it up with "Have you eaten?" She gets me a smoothie. Food to the rescue. Thank you, Tina.

I've asked them to call my husband. I'm pretty sure my ankle is broken. As I'm saying this, in rush four EMTs. They have their medical bags and are bringing in a bed on wheels. Could this get any worse? I say, "OMG, even you guys? Please tell me you didn't have the siren on." Their response "That's the best part of the job."

I now have half of Lifetime and four EMTs all working on me. *Little embarrassed here!* I'm drinking my smoothie and have cold compresses on the back of my neck. I'm feeling much better; the color comes back to my face. The EMTs offer to take me to the hospital. I want to wait for my husband. Bob finally arrives.

The paramedics put my leg in a splint and wheel me to my car. Lifetime is lit up with the flashing lights of a fire truck and ambulance. Now I'm officially mortified.

We head to the emergency. My husband tells the front desk I'm in treatment for breast cancer. He asks for a mask as flu season is in full swing. Mask on, I'm taken right back. I guess no waiting for cancer patients. I'm put in a private room.

I don't have to wait long. A PA comes in with a nurse to examine me. I'm not in too much pain and there's very little swelling. I ask him why I fainted. He told me when your body feels that kind of pain, you can faint. It goes into a fight or flight mode. It's called syncope. Well, isn't that nice? I'm a fainter on top of everything else.

He orders X-rays. Diagnosis: I've broken a non-weight-bearing bone in my ankle. I will be in an air cast for the next five to six weeks. *Oh joy.* The entire time I have radiation. Seriously, what a day.

I remind myself it could always be worse. I could have had a regular cast or even surgery, which would have been a real pain. I'll just have to create a new normal. That seems to be my life lately, creating a new normal. Can't wait to see how they get me on the table for radiation. And as far as Lifetime, I'm not sure I can show my face there again. *Never a dull moment.*

> ***Dear life, when I said, 'Can this day get any worse?'***
> ***that was a rhetorical question. Not a challenge.***
> —Anonymous

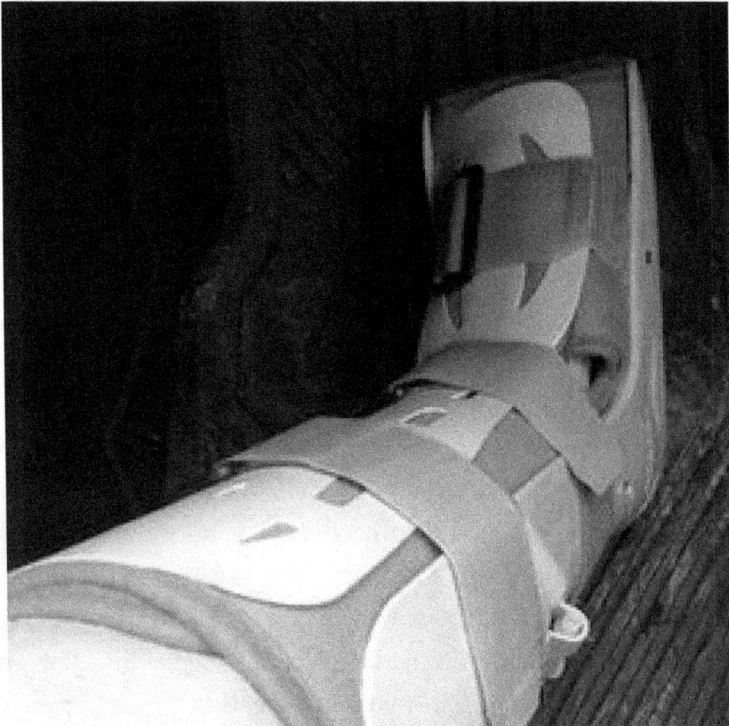

Pity Party for One
January 11th—Later That Night

I'm watching television with my foot wrapped in an Ace bandage propped up on a pillow. Exciting times for a Friday night. After a while, I decide I want to go to bed. Bob helped me up and handed me my crutches. I was still trying to figure out how to use them. While trying to maneuver, I quickly learned how **not** to use them. I fell backwards and barely missed hitting my head on the coffee table.

I wasn't hurt, but I started crying. Gut-wrenching sobs. Bob, in a panic, asks me if I've hurt anything. I'm sobbing so hard I can't talk. I finally get out No, but that's all I can say. I've *never* cried like this before; *I sound feral*. Thirty minutes later, somewhat calmer, I cry out, *"I'm so tired of this! What else, Universe?"*

I've read stories of cancer patients and how they really didn't cry until something happened that had nothing to do with their disease. The incident just triggered it. This was my trigger. I've cried during my journey but not like this. It's like a dam has burst open. I stayed on the floor for a while, while poor Bob looked on helplessly. I finally picked myself up, grabbed my crutches and limp back to my bedroom to sleep this day away.

I work hard every day to see the positive and most days I succeed. I honestly don't wake up every morning and focus on my cancer. I've just made it my new normal. While I try to stay in gratitude for my treatments, it gets overwhelming at times and breaking my ankle was one of those times. Crying gave me a release I didn't realize I needed.

> *Sometimes a good cry is just what you need to release the hurt you have built up inside.*
> —Unknown

Coming Out of the Valley Once Again
January 13th

The pity party for one continues through the weekend. I'm starting six weeks of radiation tomorrow; my left arm is swollen (I think it's lymphedema) and now this. The ramifications of having a broken ankle sink in.

Now I'm limping around, in pain, encumbered by a cast. My plan to zip in and zip out of radiation treatments is gone. I'd just started feeling somewhat normal again. I was ready to get back to life. Radiation was supposed to be easy peasy, nothing like chemo.

Now I've got to be driven, or valet park, and hobble in on crutches. Ever try walking down a hallway on crutches in a hospital gown? Yeah, trying to hold my gown together is going to be a real treat.

I'm feeling frustrated, sad, and angry. I spend most of today watching sad movies, crying at the endings. I'm halfway through my third movie when I turn off the television. I don't want to stay in sadness. I don't like feeling this way. Too much heaviness.

I hobble over and sit in my living room. I play one of my mom's Frank Sinatra albums on our new record player. Music always seems to help bring me back to a happy place. And besides, who doesn't love Old Blue Eyes?

I listen and gaze at my backyard. It looks like a winter wonderland. The music and view put me in a meditative state. I'm at peace. I feel incredibly blessed in this moment. Pure gratitude. I get to be here and take in this beauty. So what if my ankle is broken? Or I have lymphedema. I have to have radiation—big flipping deal. None of that matters because I'm here. I'M HERE. And there's nothing more precious than that. *Nothing!* My day just got brighter. Tomorrow's a new day, and I *get* to be in it. I have no complaints.

We need to appreciate how precious life is.
—Shelley Fabares

Radiation—Zapping Again

Time to Get Zapped (Radiation)
January 15th

Today, my six weeks of radiation begins. Every day at 9:36 a.m. Monday through Friday I'll be getting 'zapped.' By breaking my ankle, it's just made an easy task into a cumbersome ordeal. There's snow on the ground, so it's better if I'm driven. Walking from the parking structure to the building would be treacherous in a cast and crutches. Changing into my gown will take longer. I can't wait to see how I'm going to get on the radiation table; that ought to be a sight.

I was worried about holding my breath for 20 seconds. Could I do it? I know it doesn't sound long but having to do it on command—who knew? During the weekend, I decided to practice holding my breath so come Monday, I'd be a pro. My husband, whenever he saw me, would say, "It's no big deal; piece of cake." I'm always amazed at how the people who aren't the ones being treated know so much about how it will go for you. This morning I'll find out if he's right.

Bob drops me off at the door and I limp to the elevator. I start humming a little ditty from my favorite movie, "The Quiet Man." It's a pick-me-up kind of number. I'm feeling happy and ready to do this. I greet the receptionist, swipe my card, and am told I can go in to change after I explain about my ankle. I jokingly say, "I really didn't have enough on my plate, so I added this."

I limp into the dressing room, change into a gown, and sit in the waiting room. I pop an Altoid into my mouth. The peppermint helps me breathe easier. I'm greeted by Nancy, one of the radiation therapists, who will be with me for the next six weeks. She can't believe I've broken my ankle. "Talk about adding insult to injury," she says. "Yep," I said, "I thought I'd spice it up a bit."

I limp into the room and meet Melissa and James who will be 'zapping' me for the next six weeks. They ask me to remove my gown

177

(will I ever get over undressing in front of strangers?) They give me what looks like a green cocktail napkin to cover my chest. I immediately think, "Will it be big enough to cover these tatas?" Then, I remember I only have one tata so I'm good. Gown off, chest covered, I heave my cast up and lay down into my personal mold.

As soon as I lay my head back, *Gladys* shifts down over my eyes. I can't help but laugh at what I'm sure I look like. It made me wonder about what these people see daily. Oh, the stories they could tell.

After adjusting *Gladys*, I slip back into my mold, ready to begin. I'm told not to move; they will do the adjusting. Here's where the three tattoos come into play. They place me where they need me, lining up my tattooed dots to place my body correctly. I'm still radio station 90.5.

James hands me the mouth tube to insert. It feels awkward. I have to bite down to hold it in my mouth. I begin breathing through it. I'm getting air so I'm calm.

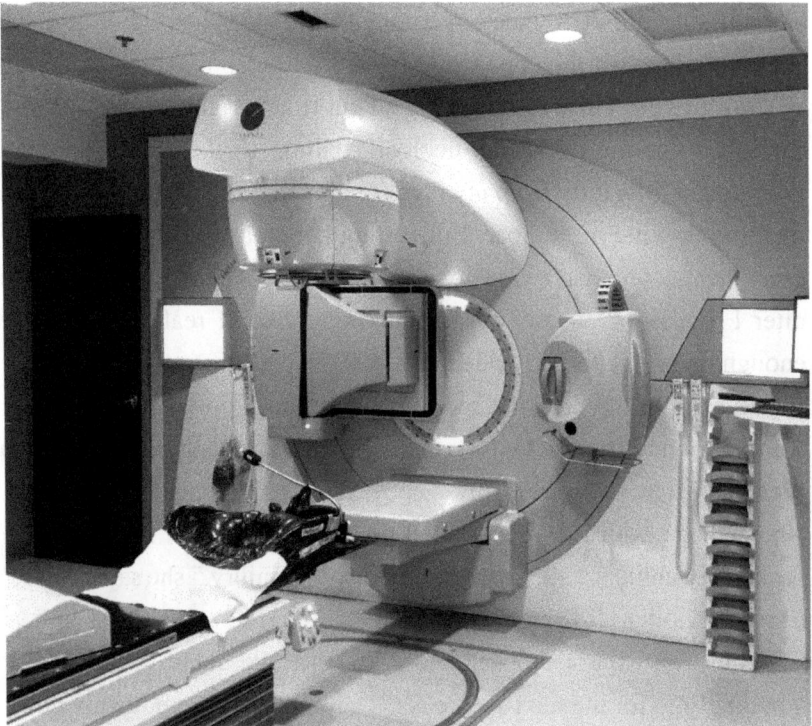

I'm given the panic button to hold which will open the airflow if I need to breathe. It makes me feel a little more in control. As I'm thinking this is doable, it happens, he plugs my nose with a clamp. I'm barely holding the panic at bay. I'm being such a wimp and we haven't even started. Calm it down, Carey. You can do this.

I take a few calming breaths. Breathing in with *gratitude*, *grace* in the pause and *grounding* when I exhale. I'm feeling peace. They check to see if I'm ready, I nod yes, and they leave the room.

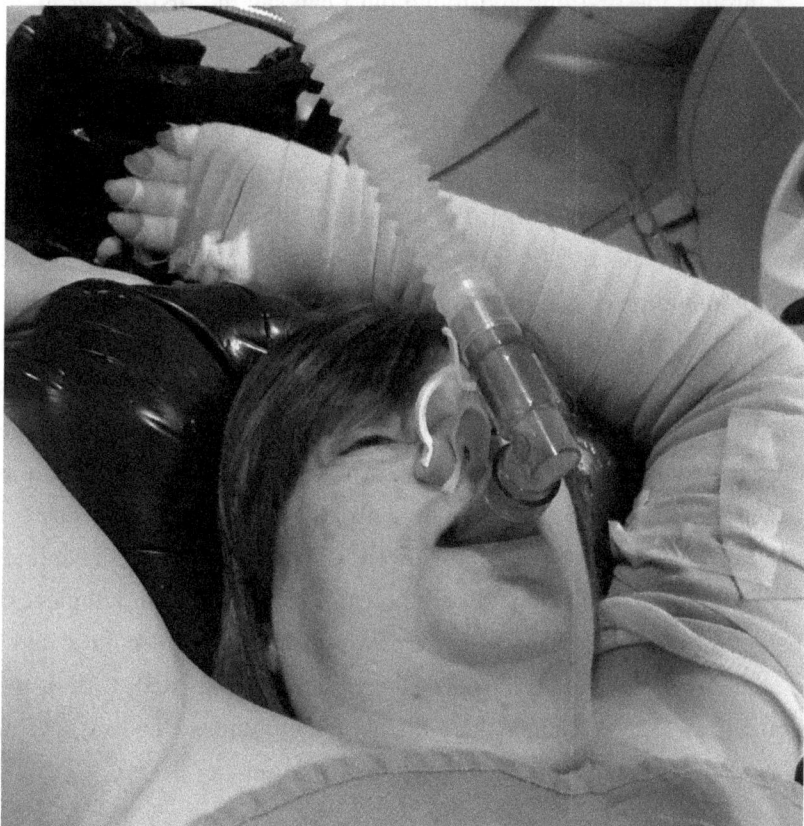

I'm alone, but I'll be able to hear them. They will talk me through each 'zap.' The machine will move around my body as it administers the beams. James comes over the speaker and asks if I'm ready to take a deep breath in. No countdown yet. They want to make sure my body is placed correctly. It is, and we begin.

Once again, James tells me to take a deep breath. As I'm still breathing in, my air supply shuts off. Wait a minute, I'm not done taking a breath. OMG, what if I don't have enough air? Am I going to have to push my panic button on the first try? Hold it in, princess.

James begins the countdown. Twenty seconds, he says. I, on the other hand, begin saying the Our Father (in my head, of course). Fifteen seconds. Me—still praying. Ten seconds—Holy Mary, Mother of God. Five seconds—Amen. Air is released. I take in a deep breath. I did it. I got through the first one and found out I can say the first prayer in 20 seconds. Five more zaps to go.

I fight the panic each time I'm told to take in a deep breath. It does start to get a little easier. I alternate between the Our Father and Hail Mary. Reciting those babies has gotten me through many tests.

The machine moves over the top half of my body, stopping in five areas. It ends directly above my head. Once finished, I'm told I can take out my mouthpiece and lay until they come in and move the machine.

While I'm getting up (with help), I want to know what they do with my mouthpiece. "Throw it away," they say. I ask if I can have mine as I have plans for it. They agree. I put on my gown and limp back to the dressing room. The procedure took a half hour. With drive time and treatment, it's a little over an hour. This will be the start of my day for the next six weeks. Onward and upward Carey, closer to the finish line.

That night when Bob and I are in bed, I bring out my mouthpiece. I have my "It's no big deal, piece of cake" man put it in his mouth, and I clamp his nose. I tell him to take a deep breath and I start the countdown. At 20 seconds, he pulls out the mouthpiece and says, "I'm so sorry, this is not a piece of cake!" Case closed.

Happiness is moving onwards and upwards.
—The Happiness Page

The Little Bastard!
January 17th

My left arm and hand were swollen. Think sausage fingers and a salami arm. (I've been married to an Italian for too long.) I could no longer wear my rings or bracelets. I went to see a lymphedema specialist. I knew about lymphedema as my mother experienced it when she had breast cancer. I figured I'd be given a sleeve and call it good.

There are two things I immediately like about this doctor. He has a great sense of humor and he's on time. After taking some measurements of both hands and arms, he tells me I have lymphedema along with cellulitis. Cellulitis? Didn't see that coming. I'm given an antibiotic for the cellulitis. He ordered physical therapy. No sleeve yet. They need to get my arm back to normal.

I will have physical therapy twice a week on Tuesday and Thursday after my radiation. It seems that the Big "C" is having fun messing with me. I hate the little bastard!

Congratulations—now I hate you.
—Unknown

Can You Say Mummy?
January 22nd

On Thursday, I met my therapist and find out I will be having a lymphatic massage along with wrapping of my arm and hand to help with my lymphedema.

I lay on a bed with my feet propped up. She gently massages different lymphatic points. This is to stimulate the rest of the lymph nodes to pick up the slack from the left side. It's painless and done quickly. It's a light massage. Now on to the wrapping. Let's put it this way, by the time she's done, my arm looks like the mummy. Thank God, it's my left arm!

Bob is videotaping the procedure as he will be the one wrapping me at home. Aquaphor is slathered on my arm, followed by a mesh sleeve. A cotton covering is wound up my arm. My arm and each finger are wrapped four times with tight Ace bandages. A piece of foam is placed on my palm. My hand and my entire left arm are wrapped from my fingers up to my shoulder.

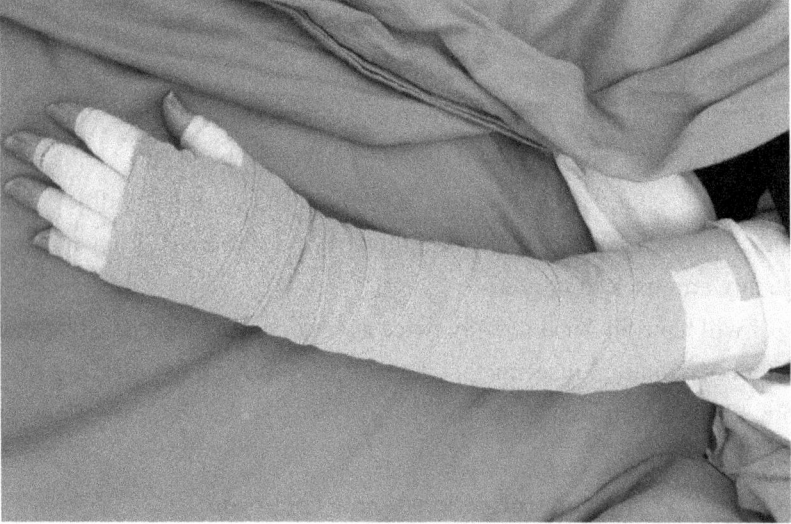

I can't move my arm or fingers. I feel stuffed like I'm in a vise. Everything is cumbersome. I will have to leave the bandages on for 48 hours. I'm only allowed to take them off when I shower. It's like we're squishing the extra liquid out of my arm. Something new to adjust to, a new normal. Thanks, Big "C".

> *My new normal is a continually getting used to new normals.*
> —Unknown

Sausage Fingers
January 24th

On Saturday, I take off my bandages. I'm happy to do it since it's been a little painful. My fingers feel like they're choking. I have so many bandages on, it will be like unwrapping King Tut. (Can't wait to roll all this stuff back up—not) I finally get everything off and look at my hand. It literally blows up before my eyes. It looks gigantic. My hand looks like the Michelin man's. Yikes!

I can push my finger into it and make a huge indentation. It's squishy. I'm concerned it's so puffy. I start to panic. Bob begins to massage my hand and arm and the swelling begins to go down. I lift my arm in the air thinking it will help. Something doesn't seem right. My arm is supposed to absorb the liquid, yet it blew up. Eventually, the swelling goes down. I refuse to wrap my hand that night. I need to give my arm a rest. Another surprise from the Big "C." Here's a surprise for you, Big "C", I'm done with surprises!

> *Is done an emotion because I feel it in my soul.*
> —Unknown

Another 'Zap'
January 26th

Broken ankle and now lymphedema. My entire left side is a mess. Cast, crutches, and now mummy arm? Can't wait to try to change into my gown for radiation, not. You've got to just laugh at it. I'm smiling when Bob takes me to radiation. I check in and get the "Are you kidding me?" Look from the receptionist. "Never a dull moment," I tell her.

Changing is a trip. I can't access my fingers. They are mummified in addition to still having neuropathy. I grab the XXXL hospital gown. It ties at the top and I figure it might be easier to get into. Slightly better, but I have a hell of a time trying to tie it. Finally, in my gown, I go sit in the waiting room.

When you receive radiation, it's the same time every day so you see the same people. You get to know your fellow patients. Carol saw me the first day I walked in with my cast and was amazed I was still smiling. When I walked in on Friday with my mummy arm, she was in shock. I tell her you've just got to laugh at this.

When Nancy comes to get me, the look on her face was priceless. I resisted the urge to put my arm up and make a mummy sound and instead just started laughing. I limp down to the radiation room and am met with the same incredulous looks from James and Melissa.

Once again resisting the urge to make a mummy sound, I finally untie my gown, but need help taking it off. Green napkin covering me, gown off, I limp on to the table. Whew! Now the concern is whether mummy arm is going to fit into my mold. Momentary panic, as I don't want anything inferring with my schedule. It fits, barely, but it fits. I'm put into position, Gladys in place, hand on the panic button and off we go. Radiation Take 2 is complete.

With my whole left side 'mummified,' I have a challenging time getting off the table. I now know what a turtle feels like when it's on its back. I get helped by James, who lends me his arm. Nancy helps me into my gown. Between being mummy wrapped and the neuropathy, I just can't tie it. Radiation angels to the rescue; they tie my gown and I'm ready to go.

When I came back from radiation my new pal, Carol, is on her way to treatment. She stopped me and said, "You know I was feeling a little down about myself and then I see you the last couple of days and think—I'm fine. If you can be so upbeat with a broken ankle and wrapped arm, I can do this." My mishaps made someone glad today. It is a good day!

> **Work miracles by setting a good example. Others will catch your spirit. The power of a good example is the greatest miracle example of all.**
> —Wilfred Peterson

Lymphedema 101
January 27th

I get to my therapy appointment and find out I was wrapped incorrectly, which is why my hand blew up. I change therapists and she does wonders. With each session and being wrapped 24/7, my arm is returning to normal.

A bonus has come out of having therapy. When a friend heard I had broken my ankle and had lymphedema, she offered to drive me to radiation and therapy. I politely turned her down as I didn't want to feel like a burden. She wouldn't take no for an answer. Barb drove me for weeks to therapy, giving Bob a much-needed break. I knew Barb but never had real one-on-one time as the only time we saw each other was at parties. During that time, I got to know a wonderful person. Cancer just gave me another gift.

At the end of six weeks of therapy, I see Dr. Riutta and my arm is no longer swollen. I don't need a sleeve—yippee! I do, however, need to wear a hand compression glove as my hand and fingers are still puffy. I will wear this on the plane to Ireland and I will bring my wrapping things in case I experience swelling. I'm good to go! The only real casualties from having lymphedema? My wedding ring is too small as my fingers have gotten bigger and I can't have my cuticles cut when I get a manicure. No big deal.

Dealing with lymphedema will be lifelong. A sunburn, heat from a sauna, bumping my arm, even a mosquito bite can make it flare up. But in the grand scheme of things, it's nothing. Just another new normal. And so it goes…

> *The key to success is often the ability to adapt.*
> —Confucious

Making it Fun…
January 28th

My husband had a job where, for the past seven years, he commuted from Detroit to Winston-Salem, North Carolina. Just before my diagnosis, he accepted another position where traveling would be limited. Looking back, the change in jobs was a godsend when going through treatment. I got to have my rock with me 24/7. (Albeit with adjustments being made with us being always together.)

Bob had to travel to Houston and was packing for his trip. He wasn't happy, grumbling under his breath and finally he said, "I hate traveling. I don't like doing this. I'm tired of it."

I will admit I wasn't in the mood for the pity party. I was going to radiation every day, my left arm wrapped like a mummy, my ankle in cast, having lymphedema therapy twice a week. My life could suck right now, but you know what? It doesn't.

Besides being grateful for being here, I'm having fun. Yes, I'm having fun while I go through treatment. I made the decision, when this first started, I would find joy. I listen to peppy, upbeat music before leaving to set my mood. I hum a little ditty while walking in to change and I smile and say hello to all I meet. I want to **enjoy** this journey.

I look at my husband and say, "Make it fun." He looks at me confused. I tell him, "Do you really think I want to go be radiated every day? Or go to therapy or limp around with a broken ankle? No, I don't, but I make it enjoyable. I have fun with it." I even dance a little walking down to radiation, the same with going to therapy for the lymphedema. I can dance in my cast like no other. Bottom line: I'm enjoying my life even though I'm going through something horrendous. I tell him, "Attitude is everything," and you know what? It is!

> *Attitude—a positive thinker does not refuse to recognize the negative, he refuses to dwell on it.*
> —Norman Vincent Peale

Friendly Competition
February 1st

When you're in treatment, you have a set appointment every day. You share the waiting room with the same patients week after week. The natural questions are asked: What are you being treated for? What type of cancer? Who's your doctor? Done with the Big "C" basics, you move on to more personal questions: family, kids, career.

It's amazing how quickly you bond. There's no judging, no wariness. You're welcomed immediately. You're part of the Club. The Club no one wants to belong to, but its members are the most incredibly caring, strong, understanding people you'd ever want to meet. They're your biggest cheerleaders. They know, more than anyone, what it feels like to be you; what you're experiencing. They simply 'get' you.

In your daily conversations, talk of treatments is done so casually. No drama just matter of fact. After a while, it's like women and childbirth. It seems like it becomes a badge of honor when discussing it with your fellow females. Each has their own 'war' story when giving birth. The same with cancer treatment.

Today, sitting with my fellow patients, we began discussing our treatment plans.

Me: *"I had a mastectomy, followed by chemo and now radiation."*

First lady: *"I had chemo, then a mastectomy and now radiation."*

Second lady: *"I had chemo, then a mastectomy followed by radiation, and once that is finished, I'm doing chemo again."*

Me: *"Ding, ding, ding! You're the winner!"*

Second lady: *"I know!"*

We all just laugh. We've just tried to one up each other about breast cancer. We are laughing together while we're treating our disease. We found our humor today. Cancer couldn't make it a sad day. The Big "C" Club members are not only caring and supportive, but they have a wicked sense of humor. If I have to be a member, I'm so glad it's with people like this.

> *A good laugh overcomes more difficulties and dissipates more dark clouds than any other one thing.*
> —Laura Ingalls Wilder

Finding the Gratitude
February 20th

On this particularly difficult day, I begin to write:

> *I have four more radiation treatments. My skin is*
> *burned and peeling. It's tight and covered with a rash*
> *in both the front and back of my chest. I can't lift my*
> *arm without pain. Sleeping is difficult at best, always*
> *trying to find a comfortable position.*

I was feeling extremely frustrated, then I read this.

> *I know that it's hard.*
> *I also know that it's temporary.*
> *It is building you.*
> *Stay strong.*
> *The storm will be over.*

And I realize this **is** temporary, and this storm **will** pass, and it has been 'building' me into a better me. My day just got brighter.

Where there are no storms, there are no rainbows.
—Matshona Dhliwayo

Ringing the Bell, One Last Time
February 23rd

I'm up early. I've been waiting for this day for eleven months. Almost an entire year. Today, I ring the bell for my final cancer treatment. I can't believe I get to say that! *Whoop! Whoop!* This dance with the Big "C" would be more invasive, treatment would take much longer. I thought my first 'dance' was challenging, looking back today, it was a piece of cake.

Chemotherapy was difficult but radiation is no walk in the park either. I have burns and a rash all over my chest. My skin is raw. I am once again feeling fatigued. But as I learned from the last time, attitude is everything.

When I was first diagnosed, 11 months seemed like a lifetime. How was I ever going to get through it? Mentally, I've been challenged like never before. I have fought daily to stay in the present moment, to stay in the now. I learned to appreciate the little things and I found humor even in horrendous situations.

I've been the recipient of love from so many people. Doctors, caregivers, family, friends, even strangers. To know everyone, I have encountered wants nothing but a positive outcome for me is humbling. Because of this, I live in gratitude.

So, after 11 long months, today I get to ring the bell signifying the end of my treatment. 9:36 a.m. can't come soon enough!

9:36 a.m.—DONE!!!

We arrive early as I'm beyond excited to finish treatment. I've had 'boob' cake pops made to pass out to everyone who's cared for me during my time here. I begin to pass them out and receive smiles from everyone. Dr. Chen's intern says, "Well this is a first, I've got to take a picture of these."

I gladly walk back to the changing room and quickly get ready for the final zap. I'm walking on clouds, well limping on clouds, but I'm floating with happiness. I receive hugs from my radiation angels, take pictures and lay down for one last zap. Laying there for the last time, I'm overcome with emotions. I'm both happy and sad. Happiness this grueling journey is over and some sadness it even happened. But most of all I'm filled with immense gratitude. *I'm here! I survived!*

It's time to ring the bell. Bob is the only one with me. Riley was still in school, and Nick and Anthony were working. I originally thought I wanted a cast of thousands with me to celebrate. But in the end, it was just the two of us ringing the bell and it was simply perfect.

We had navigated this journey together. We held each other up, laughed at the absurdities, cried at the frustrations, and at the end of each day, we were thankful for that day. We had climbed the highest mountain **together**.

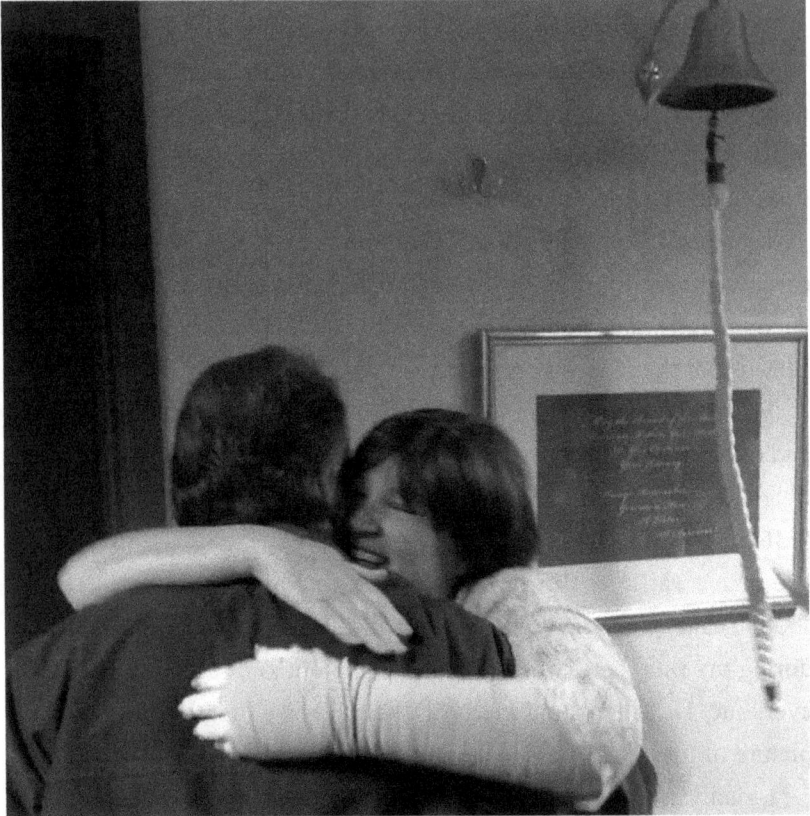

Today when I rang the bell, I did so with my biggest supporter, my best friend, my husband. We hugged and cried, but this time it was happy tears. We were done. No more treatments. Let the healing begin. *It is a great, great day!*

> **Life is like a mountain, hard to climb, but worth the amazing view from the top.**
> —Unknown

Burn, Baby, Burn!
February 26th

I'm singing "Disco Inferno" in my head as I write this—"Burn, baby, burn." Since I also had cancer in my skin, they needed to adjust my treatment. I would receive regular radiation (if there is such a thing) and then halfway through they would place a wet towel on my chest for the next part of the treatment. This towel would simulate a layer of skin. It's called a bolus treatment. This would allow the radiation to penetrate deeper into my skin. *Oh joy!*

I've watched my skin diligently. I was told by many people outside the medical field to moisturize. When mentioning this to the staff, I was told an emphatic NO. Studies have shown it doesn't help and could make it worse. No moisturizing for me. Every Thursday, when meeting with Dr. Chen, my mantra was the same: *Don't burn me.*

I'm nearing the end of my six weeks of treatment, and it's happened. I'm burned. My skin is raw, and I'm uncomfortable. Talking with Bev, my nurse, she said it will get worse for about two weeks after treatment. *Great.* My burn is going to get worse? *Enough is enough, people.*

She gives me an astringent with gauze. I'm to apply this several times a day to help dry up the area. If my skin starts oozing or I have a fever, I'm to call her. This just got serious. What am I in for? I kept hearing from everyone that radiation was a breeze compared to chemo. While it may be true, radiation isn't a picnic, either. I was being radiated 5 days a week for six weeks. I'm feeling fatigued and severely burned. It really hurts and I'm in pain. My skin is exposed and wet in some spots. Wearing clothes is brutal, I can't wear a bra.

I walk with my left arm up in the air because my skin is so raw. Forget getting into a comfortable position to sleep. I try to prop my arm up on a pillow to keep from touching the area. When sleeping, I wear a huge shirt only covering my right side, leaving my left side clothing free. *(Thinking out loud here, why did I even bother with wearing anything?)* I apply astringent right before I go to sleep in the hopes of drying my skin.

I have a fan attached to my iPhone and I'm using it constantly on the area to help my skin dry. I've had a **miserable** few days. This is not easy. I'm pretty sure all the people who told me radiation was a breeze never had it before. Chemo was fatigue and nausea. This, in comparison, is painful.

Having the radiation, no big deal. The aftereffects, huge deal. But as with anything, slowly but surely, I'm beginning to heal. The wet areas are drying up. The burned skin is flaking off and my skin is beginning to look better.

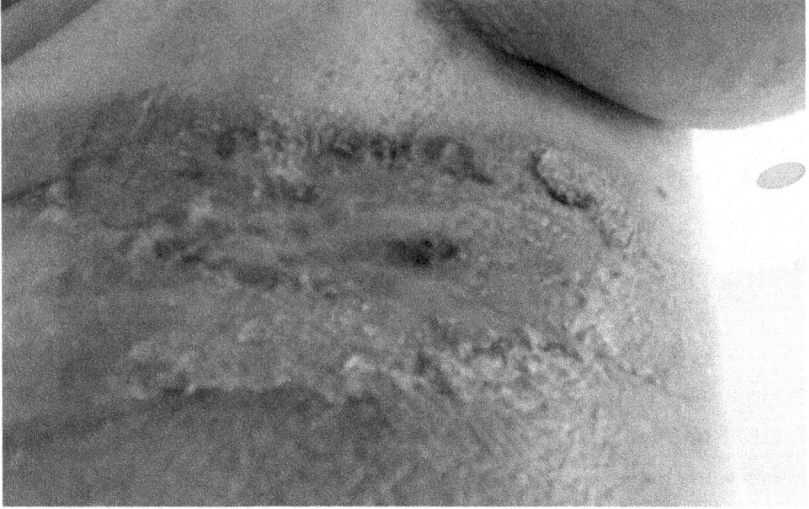

It takes a few weeks, but my skin is healed. Life is starting to return to my new normal. Looking back, I don't know why I was so naïve to think I wouldn't burn as I roast just looking at the sun. I was told at my radiation orientation there was the possibility of it happening. I knew the score going in. I was just so convinced it was going to be so much easier than chemo that I didn't entertain the thought that it could be difficult. Another surprise from cancer.

It's done—treatment is complete. So what if I'm burned? I'm here and all the pain and fatigue were worth it. I went through a little bit of hell, but I survived, and it feels fantastic to be able to say that!

> *Life is not about waiting for the storms to pass. It's*
> *about learning how to dance in the rain.*
> —Vivian Greene

LIFE POST CANCER

A New Chapter

Can You Say Wolfman?
March 1st

I couldn't wait for my hair to begin growing. I desperately wanted my eyebrows and eyelashes back. Ever hear the saying, *"Be careful what you wish for"*? Well, I got my wish. My hair is growing back—everywhere. My eyebrows, it seems, are taking their job of growing back very seriously. It's like they feel they have to make up for lost time. They're growing into a shape I've never seen before. Oh wait, I've seen these eyebrows before, on *Wolfman!*

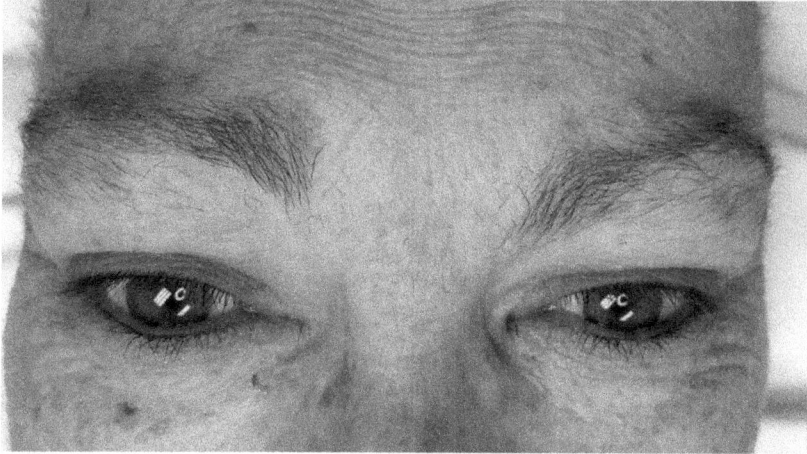

Seriously, my eyebrows are coming in thick, black, and bushy. These new eyebrows seem to start at the inside of my eye and make a huge crescent. They're a half inch wide for God's sake. I even have hair at the base of my eyes. Really? A positive: My eyelashes are coming in tremendously thick—*Whoop! Whoop!*

The hair on my head is growing in. My first growth was white and very fine. It was then followed by jet black sprouts. These sprouts were itchy. The itching has stopped and now I have a downy-like feel to my hair. It's incredibly soft and salt and pepper. Not so sure I like the salt and pepper, but I've got hair growing. *Score.*

I stopped by to see Debbie, my hairdresser, last week. I wanted to show her my hair progress and my Wolfman eyebrows. She tells me when my hair grows in a little more, she can stain it to make it look thicker. Yippee, the news is getting better. Goodbye, white hair.

She offers to wax my eyebrows and upper lip (yes, I have hair there). Yay! Something normal. She waxes and shapes my eyebrows. My upper lip next. (*Ouch*) I finally have enough hair, in some places, that needs to be removed. How about that?

Now being fair (let's call a spade a spade: I'm pale, white, translucent), my skin where she's removed the hair is bright red. Debbie is worried, she's done some damage. No, I tell her, it's just my skin. What I don't tell her is I'm thrilled to have my skin turn red. I won't mind people seeing it, even though prior to the Big "C", I would have been trying to cover it up. No, this to me, means life is returning to normal. My upper lip and eyebrows are red because I had hair to remove. *I had hair!* I'll deal with having redness because it's one step back to my life.

> **It looks like we're starting to get back to normal.**
> —Steve Coleman

Now What?
March 12th

I had my last radiation treatment three weeks ago. This week is the first week since my diagnosis I don't have an appointment. Eleven months of weekly doctor appointments, poking and prodding, examinations, surgeries, chemotherapy, radiation, physical therapy. I've been 'doing' cancer for almost a year.

A year of my life journeying through the Big "C". All treatments are completed. I'm now going into maintenance mode. I'll be seeing my doctors periodically through the year for checkups.

Now what? What do I do now? I've been doing cancer for so long, I'm not sure what to do with myself. I don't have to plan my week around appointments. I no longer have to drive to Beaumont; I'm done with hospitals. I'm done with examinations. No more hospital gowns. Better yet, I don't have to take off my hospital gown in front of any more people. *Score! I'm done with all of that.* And while I'm elated to be done with treatment, I'm feeling a little lost.

I was talking to my husband about it, and he said something that resonated with me. *"You've been in fight mode for almost a year."* He was right. I got a seat on the Big "C" roller coaster, and it's been a wild ride ever since. The peaks and valleys, twists, and turns, kept me on my toes. I was in survival mode. High alert.

I've survived the storm and as Bob and I joke to each other on particularly difficult days, *"We live to fight another day."* I'm alive. There are still days where I feel a little shell-shocked and say, *"Did that just happen?"* I'm slowly beginning to realize I no longer need to be on high alert. I can breathe a little easier. I remind myself to stay present.

I am creating another new normal. A life that doesn't have to revolve around cancer. A life that gets to create new memories, experience new adventures and challenges and just *be*. Cancer will always be a part of who I am, but it will no longer consume me. It will just be another experience in my life.

It's now time to decompress, relax, build up my strength and let myself heal. I think I'm putting too much pressure on myself. At times, I feel I've been in a cocoon for a year, and I've got to hurry up and make up for lost time, that I need to be doing something all the time. And what I've just realized is I don't have to do a thing; go with the flow. Just be. When the time is right, I'll know what my next step should be, so for now, I'll just be and take in the gratitude of another day.

> ***It's okay to stop and just be.***
> —Unknown

Estelle and my Wig
March 27th

My brother, Ritchie, and his wife, Pat, have "Tuesday night dinner" which his entire family attends. This tradition has been in place for years. This is one of the highlights of the week for my mom. Since I was with her all day for shopping and appointments, we went together.

Several of us were in the family room while waiting for dinner. Estelle, who's four, stopped playing and came and sat next to me on the couch. With a very serious expression, she put her little hand on my arm and said, "Aunt Carey, are you all done being sick?" I smiled and said, "Yep, I'm all better." She kept staring at me and then said, "Is that a wig you're wearing?" I replied, "Why, yes, it is. Do you want to see what's underneath?" She looked a little pensive at first then said, "Yes."

There were a few people around me, so I asked if they minded if I took off my wig. Estelle got very serious and said, "Maybe we should go into the other room." How sweet of her to think of my feelings. "No, it's alright to do it here," I replied. I asked her if she wanted to take it off. She promptly said, "No." I pulled off my wig. Estelle looked at me in surprise and immediately said, "Quick! Quick! Put it back on." I guess I didn't look that great without my wig. (Harper, also four, obviously didn't notice my look as she put it on and ran to show her mother—lol!) Once I had Gladys back in place Estelle looked at me and said, "Much, much better, Aunt Carey." Don't you just love the honesty of children?

> *Pretty much all the honest truth telling in the world is done by children*
> —Oliver Wendell Holmes

Cancer Gave Me an Incredible Gift
April 13th

Riley is obtaining her Bachelor of Fine Arts (BFA) in dance from Western Michigan University. As part of her program, she has to choreograph a 7- to 10-minute piece as her graduating presentation. She is responsible for choreography, lighting, staging, costumes, auditions; the full gamut.

In addition to the performance, she must also write a paper on the concept of her dance, what she is trying to convey in her piece, why she chose the music and a detailed account of the meaning behind every movement in the dance. It is a huge undertaking.

The BFA candidates submit their theme for their dance in the fall; the performance is in April. When I ask Riley what her theme is going to be, she tells me she's not ready to share.

Throughout the next months, I watched my daughter shed blood, sweat and tears to complete her piece. She's never been a choreographer or had a desire to be one. She just wants to dance. There were a few nights where there were tears and frustration, but when all was said and done, she found out she was a choreographer. She was extremely proud of herself and the piece she created.

She was still tight-lipped about the theme but said she was getting compliments from everyone who had seen the piece. I was extremely excited to see it.

We arrive for the BFA Graduating Presentations, with Nick and Molly, and go to our seats. While we're waiting for the show to begin one of the ushers asks if I'm Riley's mom. "Yes," I reply. "This is for you to read before the show starts. It's from Riley."

A woman behind me must know what's up as she taps me on the shoulder and says you may want to wait to read that if you don't want the waterworks to start. *OK then, words I wasn't expecting.*

I open and read this:

Dear Mom,

Coming into my senior year, I had a clear vision of what I wanted my Graduating Presentation to be about. I think you have an idea by now. . . For my piece I wanted to show your pure strength, gratitude and perseverance. To me, my entire life you have been exactly that, even when times were tough for you. When we got the news of your second diagnosis with breast cancer, our worlds turned upside down. This is something we all never thought would happen again. Seeing you go through this not once, but twice, was most definitely life-altering.

The day of your surgery to the day I came home from Europe are memories that will always stick with me. It was difficult to comprehend the changes you were going to face, but I was more than ready to tackle them with you. You showed me through these difficult times there is always gratitude and love. Like you always say, this is life-changing not life-taking. Because of your positive attitude and strength throughout this whole journey, I truly believe it. Nothing can tear you down, not even the Big "C".

My inspiration for my piece is you, Mom. And although this is a heavy topic, I did not want to focus on the dark side. I wanted to show your journey and how there are ups and downs, and within those dark moments there is always gratitude and love. I wanted to focus on when there are hard days, you are constantly showing strength. And that overall, there is healing, love and hope. Thank you for being my role model. Thank you for being my best friend. Thank you for being my mom.

I love you,
Riley

I'm speechless and yes, the waterworks begin. My daughter dedicated her dance to my journey. Something so fresh and raw in her life and she wanted to depict what it meant to her. Not only did she show what she learned from our experience, she didn't focus on the negative. She wanted to convey that even in the journey with the Big "C", *there is* hope, healing and love.

I have just witnessed my daughter learn an incredible life lesson. She got it. She understood what I'm trying to *live*. Yes, cancer sucks, but look at the incredible gift it just gave me. A dance which beautifully shows my journey and an amazing daughter who loves me so much she dedicated her Graduating Presentation to me. She understands how being in gratitude and staying positive are everything. I'm feeling blessed, humbled, surprised, grateful, happy all rolled into one. If I'm crying now, how am I going to make it through her number?

The show begins. Each number is unique, showing the dancer's personality, with a theme which means something to them. It's time for her number and it doesn't disappoint. It's beautiful, heartbreaking, and joyous. It portrayed hope, healing, and love. I cry through most of it, praying it's on video so I can watch it again when my eyes aren't so blurry. When it's done, she gets a standing ovation. All the dancers are crying; the piece has also moved them.

While waiting for Riley, I speak with her ballet professor and mentor for this piece. She hugs me for a long time and with tears in her eyes, she says, "Your daughter did a phenomenal job. I tried to talk her out of this theme as it was so fresh and raw and she stood steadfast. Her choreography depicted it beautifully."

She went on to tell me my daughter didn't tell any of her professors until right before the presentations about my illness. After they learned of my diagnosis, they told her they were in awe of her professionalism and demeanor. They admired her strength. She never missed a class or an assignment and was always present. I am once again speechless. I'm a parent so I naturally think my children are amazing (it comes with the territory), but tonight I am truly in awe of my daughter.

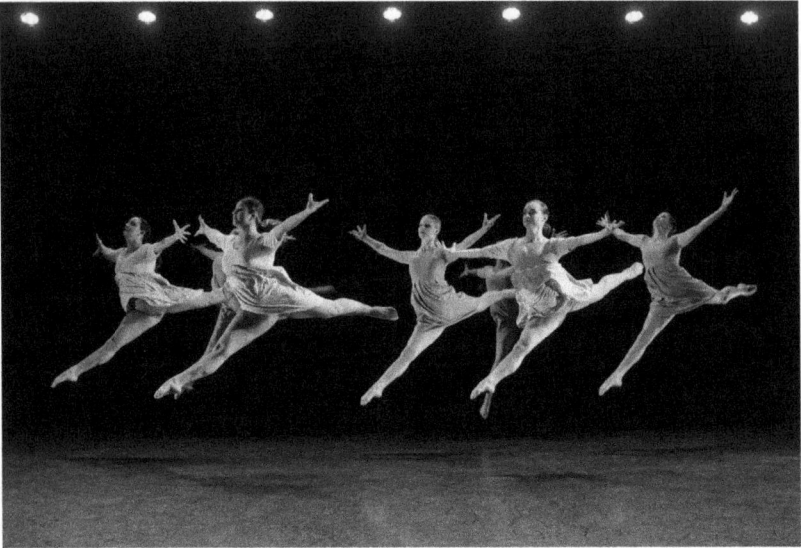

Picture courtesy of A. Deran Photography.

What she created through her grief and how she handled herself throughout my journey touches my soul. It's *so hard* to be a parent with cancer. You are trying to work through so many of your own emotions, but it can't just be about you, you have children. You have responsibilities, you can't walk away.

You want to help them process their feelings; ease their worry and pain. You hope by watching you they can see struggles are surmountable. My daughter showed me that tonight. She has learned the importance of being positive and having gratitude; how she can focus and grow through pain. I have a feeling of peace tonight as I realize Riley is becoming a compassionate, self-assured woman. One who can tackle what life throws at her and handle it with a grace beyond her years. Tonight, cancer gave me a gift I'll always treasure.

> **The greatest gifts are not wrapped in paper but in love.**
> **—Unknown**

Picking Lilies
May 26th

I picked lily of the valley from my garden this morning. I savored the moment. I took in the breathtaking smell and thought back to this time last year when I was weeding and picking flowers like a madwoman to keep my mind busy.

Today, when I was out picking flowers, I embraced the moment. The sun was out, everything was green, the air smelled like lilies, birds were chirping and there was peace.

I'm in gratitude as I write this. The storm is over. It's a sunny day. I got to pick flowers and I'm cancer free. Life is continuing to move forward. Another season is here, and I get to embrace it. Pure joy!

> *If we never had any storms, we couldn't appreciate the sunshine.*
> —Dale Evans

Ireland—A Dream Come True
June 1st – 9th

As our trip approached, I realized we were leaving on the one-year anniversary of my mastectomy. How perfect to leave on our dream trip on that date.

Where do I begin? Our trip was perfect. I'm not exaggerating when I say that. It **was** perfect. We all had the trip of a lifetime. We laughed, cried, explored, and enjoyed being a family again. We forgot about cancer, celebrated life, and were grateful to be with each other.

Our driver, James Clifford, was the ultimate host. Nice Irish smile, charming blue eyes, and a keen intelligence. I think he was a gift to us. He said, after the second day, he was getting a good read on us. He got us, he truly did. James caught on to Anthony's love of cars, Riley's love of sheep and our family's love of abandoned castles and ruins. He knew we weren't into the tourist traps but were more into seeing and experiencing the nature of Ireland.

We began in Dublin and experienced the famed Temple Bar area where we witnessed how the Irish do stag and hen parties (bachelor and bachelorette parties). We wandered around the city and enjoyed the sites. It was a great start to our trip.

From there, we stayed in Galway, Ennis, Killarney and Kinsale. James took us to small towns and out-of-the-way spots that took our breath away. We saw the Cliffs of Moher by boat in the fog. It was eerily magical. We stayed in Dromoland Castle, an elegant 5-star hotel with opulence everywhere. It was on my bucket list to stay in a castle, and it lived up to the hype.

We were riding in the coach one day and the kids were in the back laughing and joking with each other. Bob and I looked at each other with tears in our eyes and smiled. We agreed it was simply perfect. How long had it been since we heard genuine laughter? We were all feeling a little lighter. This was a trip for fun; cancer wasn't allowed.

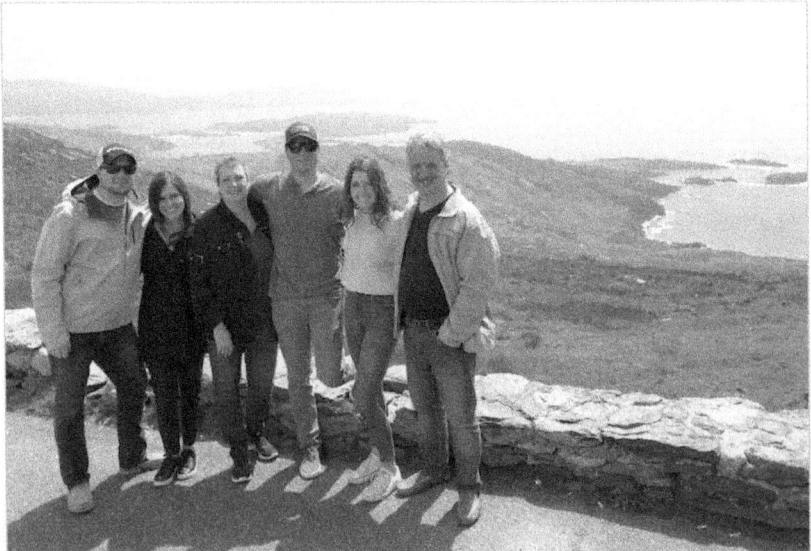

I watched all of us bring out our inner child as we climbed and explored all the castles and ruins. Even the "slow man," Nick, was jumping and climbing. It's like we'd been in a holding pattern for the last year, and we were finally emerging out of the fog. We just loved having fun. One of our favorite memories was walking the beach. We were acting like kids, throwing stones, putting our feet in the water, running from waves. We were joyous together.

Ireland was truly magical. It was the perfect way to end the journey of last year. The people were friendly, the landscape was breathtaking, the food was terrific, we had perfect weather (no rain, sunny and in the 70s), but it was being together for a week which made it so special.

We needed this trip to reconnect without having cancer looming over us. We celebrated us as a family and realized once again what we mean to each other, how much we enjoy each other's company. There will be more trips in the future, but this one will always hold a special place in my heart. We were saying goodbye to the Big "C" and hello to a brand-new future for all of us.

> *And suddenly you know... it's time to start something new and trust the magic of new beginnings.*
> —Unknown

Cancer—A Universal Word
June 9th

Cancer. The word is universal. When we were returning from Ireland, we had a connecting flight in Amsterdam. We only had 30 minutes between flights. Our plane landed and we were off and running. Weaving our way through the crowded airport, we saw on the screen our flight was boarding. Can you say panic?

While we were running, I was busy trying to get out our passports. I had the four of ours, Nick and Molly had their own. We finally get to the gate. Bob, Anthony, Riley, and I are standing while the agent looks at our boarding passes along with our passports. He takes his time making sure each passport picture matches each person.

My passport is last. He looks at it and then me, he does this three times. I finally laugh, point to my head, and say the universal word—*cancer*. "Ahh," he says in broken English. "All good, I hope?" I say, "Yes, all good!" He waves us on and wishes me well.

We board the plane to head home. When I'm sitting, I laugh about my encounter with the agent, and I get a little sad at the same time. Smiling once again because cancer gave me a laugh but also sad because the whole world knows cancer.

> *Cancer is something that touches everyone's lives.*
> —Ellen Pompeo

Musings

Angels on Earth

I believe there are people on Earth who were born to heal souls. Selfless beings whose only mission is to bring love and healing. I think about my doctors: Dr. Deborah Ruark, my breast surgeon; Dr. Yousef Hanna, my oncologist; Dr. Michael Walker, my naturopath oncologist, and Dr. Peter Chen, my radiation oncologist. They work every day with patients who are living their worst fear—Cancer.

Think about it. You know the information you're going to give someone is going to change their world. You witness your patient's reactions to facing their mortality. They're realizing life has just changed drastically and it will never be quite the same. You're the General leading the charge in their battle to stay alive. They look to you to help them navigate the nightmare they're in. You are their hope against the Big "C". What an incredible burden to shoulder. Yet they do so daily.

They treat your cancer to ensure you have a fighting chance. Their goal is to make this unpleasant journey as manageable as possible. All my doctors were extremely professional, knowledgeable, and compassionate. I never felt intimidated or disrespected. I felt cared for. *"The good physician treats the disease; the great physician treats the patient with the disease."* —Sir William Osler

The same could be said of all the hospital personnel I encountered. Every PA, nurse advocate, resident, chemo nurse and radiation tech. The list is endless. Every single person I came across on this journey showed me nothing but kindness. From hugs to simple things like tying my hospital gown, I was treated with compassion. Everyone is in your corner. They want you to have a positive journey.

People who choose to go into these types of careers have a special calling. They see you at your most vulnerable, know you're petrified of what the future brings, and work hard to give you peace. It can be overwhelmingly emotional. Working around cancer can be incredibly depressing, yet they show up every day working to give each patient a fighting chance. I am thankful for every one of my caregivers. I am here today because of them. They are my proof that there are angels on Earth.

> *I've seen and met angels in the disguise of ordinary people living ordinary lives.*
> —Tracy Chapman

Things You Should Never Say to a Cancer Patient

Navigating cancer is difficult, but when insensitive people say ignorant things to you, it hurts. Until you have cancer, you have no idea what it's like. *"Walk in someone else's shoes."* I know most people mean well and have your best interests at heart, but honestly, I wonder if they truly think before they speak. Below are some things *not* to say to someone who has cancer:

Just realize you're going to have a terrible year. I refuse to go there. This journey will give me many gifts and abundant love.

Know you're going to physically feel terrible. Once again, I refuse to go there.

What's your success rate? Makes me feel like you're asking me if I'm going to die.

Are you sorry you did a clinical trial the last time? I mean maybe it didn't catch it all. I won't look back, only forward.

It could be a worse cancer. Cancer is cancer no matter what type.

My friend had cancer and had a terrible time with it. While I empathize, I don't want to hear other people's horror stories.

Let me tell you about my experience. Truly, not to diminish your journey, but everyone experiences it differently. Reminds me of hearing childbirth stories. They scared me more than they helped me.

You talked or saw other people and not me? I care about you, I love you, but don't want the pressure of that statement.

You're so brave. I'm not brave. I'm just being me. I'm navigating this the only way I know how.

Are you sure you have the right doctors/treatment? Trust my judgment. This isn't my first rodeo.

What you're going through is just textbook. There is nothing 'textbook' about cancer. Everyone is unique and to belittle someone's care as just as everyone else's is demeaning. Textbook. What does that mean anyway?

Are you sorry you didn't have your breast removed the first time you had cancer? Asked by a technician one day. Not even dignifying that with a response.

And my all-time favorite:

Why don't you stop the façade of being so positive? I will admit that one really wounded my heart especially since it came from someone close to me. Staying on the bright side is what gets me through this journey. The dark side doesn't serve you. And quite frankly, I don't know any other way to be. I prefer to look at life in gratitude. Yes, I have down days, but I refuse to stay there. I see the glass as half full. Always have, always will. In fact, the glass is refillable.

> *Wise men speak because they have something to say;*
> *fools because they have to say something.*
> —Plato

Side Effects
(Because Treatment Isn't Enough)

Treating cancer is physically debilitating. The one constant is the side effects. At times, it seemed they were worse than the actual treatment. Every time I went for a consult, I would be given list of the possible adverse reactions. It reminded me of the commercials on television. They tell you about the drug, then spend most of the commercial listing the side effects. I read this in a meme, *"Why are there never any good side effects? Just once I'd like to read a medication bottle that says, 'May cause extreme sexiness.'"* I wish!

Keeping the side effects at bay became a full-time job. The vitamins and medications I took every day filled a large basket. I kept a spreadsheet which listed the drugs and next to each drug, what I needed to take or do to counteract the negative effects.

Pain medication could cause constipation, so every night before going to bed, I'd take a stool softener. I wouldn't let anyone give me that pill, especially Bob. Nope, not letting that happen again!

Two pillows shaped like hearts were a godsend. I placed them under my arms post-surgery. They kept my arms away from my body. *Best invention ever.* Before my surgery, we bought a La-Z-Boy to keep my body cocooned when sleeping. I made sure to wear loose clothing which was easy to remove. Using Arnica cream regularly on my post-surgery scars helped with wound healing, bruising, and discoloration.

During the first four rounds of chemo, I would set an alarm for 4 a.m. and take my anti-nausea meds to stay on top of a six-hour schedule. I was rotating two different drugs and taking Marinol to keep the nausea at bay.

The first round of chemo, I loved Vernors. It was the one thing that tasted great. When I was prepping for my second chemo, I stocked up on it. Lo and behold, after round two I couldn't stand the taste. Now root beer was my favorite. Bob and I would have date nights at the A&W. There is nothing better than a cold root beer in a glass mug. (*Relish the small things.*)

Toward the end of the four rounds of A/C, I lost my sense of taste. It felt like eating texture instead of flavors. Between the nausea and having no taste buds eating was a chore. My naturopath oncologist had recommended following a Mediterranean diet. Lucky for me one of the things I did like was hummus. Olives and cheese were also favorites, so I became the charcuterie queen.

It was important for me to drink two liters of water a day. Some days it was a struggle as everything tasted like chemicals. Eating popsicles was a good alternative. I constantly had a mini Altoid in my mouth. The peppermint helped, so I would take them with me to the pool to pop one in mid workout. Swimming kept my energy levels up.

Acupuncture reduced the nausea. I swished Biotene four times a day to prevent mouth sores from developing. Aromatherapy diffusers helped with my heighten sense of smell. Eucalyptus being my go-to scent. Meditating daily kept me calm.

I bought wigs, hats, and scarves to cover my bald head. I tried unsuccessfully to keep my eyebrows by applying ESS twice a day.

When my skin burned from the radiation, I used Aquaphor and an astringent. I dutifully wrapped my arm for the lymphedema and made sure to never miss an appointment for therapy.

As I'm reading this over to check for errors, I'm shaking my head in wonder. I sometimes forget all the things I did to keep the side effects at bay. It **was** a full-time job. Treating cancer isn't the actual treatments, it's surviving the side effects. Ain't that the truth!

Recovery is a process. It takes time, it takes patience, it takes everything you've got.
—Unknown

Final Thoughts

I didn't want cancer once, let alone twice, but nevertheless, the universe put me on the Big "C" journey. Both journeys were filled with peaks and valleys. I experienced joy and sadness. Both brought pain, physically and mentally. It has changed me. How could it not? Cancer does that. It shoves your mortality in your face, comes at you with everything it has, strips you down to the basics. You go into complete survival mode.

Staying present and keeping a mantra of 'temporary' helps maintain a positive attitude. You must reach for gratitude. Even on days when you are so sick and discouraged, despite it all, you are still here, alive. Find your humor, as laughter makes most things 'lighter.' It's so simple, but it's those simple things which help you maintain a sense of sanity.

Physically, I had two lumpectomies and had my breast surgically removed. I went through 16 rounds of grueling chemotherapy with all the lovely side effects. (Loss of hair, debilitating nausea, fatigue.) I can't count how many times I've been poked and prodded. I had no sense of taste for 10 months, experienced neuropathy in my fingers and toes. I developed lymphedema.

My body has been through radiation twice, once through a clinical trial and another with traditional treatment, getting 'zapped' every day for 6 weeks. I had severe burns over my chest along with crippling fatigue. Oh, and then non-cancer related, I broke my ankle. My body and my mind have been through hell—literally.

Like any challenge in life, the Big "C" has given me powerful lessons:

- I learned struggles develop strength.
- The right attitude helps one get through anything.
- Being positive *always* wins over negativity.
- Finding gratitude every day can bring peace, even amid chaos.
- And with humor comes joy.

All these lessons helped me live my life, not the disease. I pray it does the same for you.

Will the Big "C" always be with me? Probably. Every time I feel a twitch or ache, I'll wonder, *is it back*? But, for the most part, it is a distant memory, one stored in the back of my mind brought out occasionally, as a gentle reminder I journeyed with cancer and found myself in the process.

Writing about my journeys made me vulnerable to sharing my thoughts and feelings. It was difficult to let people see you, warts, and all. I was not sure how I would be received. Would I share TMI? What I found from my family and friends was understanding and encouragement. The abundant love and support from them overwhelmed and humbled me. This is the true gift that has come from me having cancer. I have been given **love**. *When you have love, you have hope.* Is there anything more beautiful than that?

And lastly, laughing is, and will always be, the best form of medicine. To quote my idol, Erma Bombeck, *"Laughter rises out of tragedy when you need it most and rewards you for your courage."* May you always find the laughter.

Love and light,

Carey

> *And once the storm is over, you won't remember how you made it through, how you managed to survive. You won't even be sure, whether the storm is really over. But one thing is certain. When you come out of the storm, you won't be the same person who walked in. That's what this storm's all about.*
> —Haruki Murakami

All the best on your journey.

From my family to yours.

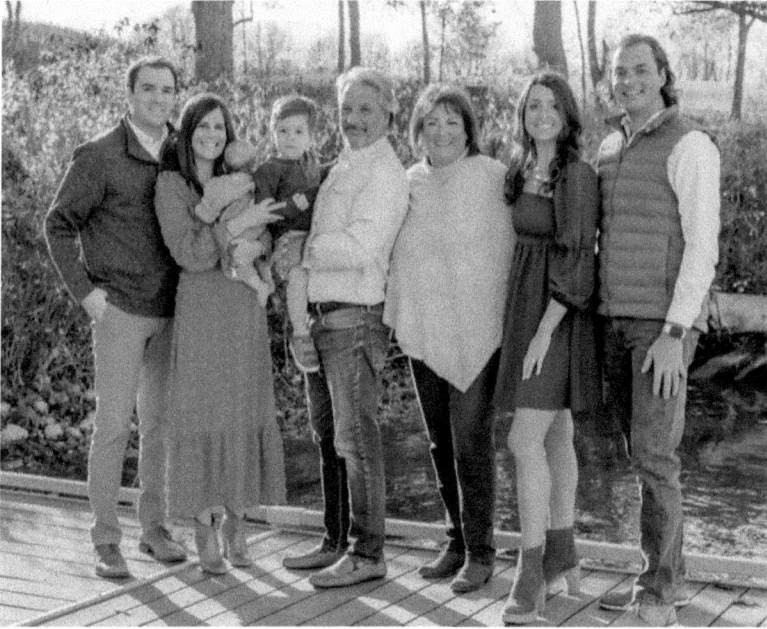

About the Author

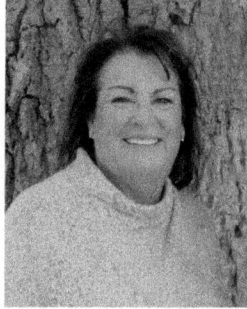

Carey Teets Cornacchini is a two-time breast cancer survivor who is living her best life on Lake Oakland in Michigan with her husband, Bob and cockapoo, Evie (weak Covid moment). Journaling and blogging helped her cope with the wild ride. Writing about her cancer journey allowed Carey to face, and ultimately release, her fears, and frustrations. While claiming she's not a writer, family, friends, and readers have said otherwise. After overwhelmingly positive reviews, and with much encouragement (like a lot!), Carey decided to share her journey in book form so others can know treating cancer can be an experience filled with love, hope, and even humor. Mother to three fantastic (most times) children, Nick, Anthony, and Riley. She is ecstatic to be CeCe. (Notice she didn't say grandmother.) To quote her idol Erma Bombeck, *"Grandparenthood is one of life's rewards for surviving your own children."* She enjoys traveling, cooking, reading, and watching old movies (TCM addict). She especially loves lake living and all it entails. Life is all about adventure and she's grabbing it whenever she can.

To learn more, please visit her website: **SavingTeets.com**

Additional Materials & Resources

Access your Additional Materials & Resources
referenced throughout this book at
SavingTeets.com/bookbonus

www.ingramcontent.com/pod-product-compliance
Lightning Source LLC
Chambersburg PA
CBHW062127020426
42335CB00013B/1128